THE BOWEN TECHNIQUE

THE BOWEN TECHNIQUE

Julian Baker

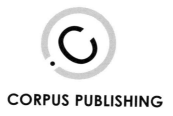

CORPUS PUBLISHING

© Corpus Publishing Limited 2001

First published in 2001. Reprinted with additions in 2002 by
Corpus Publishing Limited
4/5 The Marina Harbour Road Lydney Gloucestershire United Kingdom GL15 5ET

Author's note

The anatomy used in this book is for guidance only and no claim regarding accuracy is given. Similarly where directions and words are used, this is to give an opportunity for the reader to obtain independent reference. I have used throughout the word client, rather than patient. The word 'Patient', in my view, implies an element of clinical control and within the confines of The Bowen Technique is not something that is desirable or sought. I have generally spoken of 'The Therapist' but will on occasion refer to him or her. No express meaning or implication is meant.

Disclaimer

This publication is intended as an informational guide. The techniques described are a supplement, and not a substitute for professional tuition. Whilst the information herein is supplied in good faith, no responsibility is taken by either the publisher or the author for any damage, injury or loss, however caused, which may arise from the use of the information provided.

British Library Cataloguing in Publication Data
A CIP record for this book is available from the British Library
ISBN 1 903333 06 7

Text and Cover Design Sara Howell
Cartoons Bryan Davies
Drawings Amanda Williams
Printed and bound in Great Britain by Bell & Bain Ltd., Glasgow

Contents

A Message from Tom Bowen's Daughters

We were delighted to each receive a copy of Julian's book. We thought that here at last was someone who recognised the genius of the man Tom Bowen, but also acknowledged he had a family who sacrificed time with their father so he could help others. We should say that we know little in the way of detail about his technique, but just know it works, having had some very positive results when we have needed his therapy.

Our father could have been a very wealthy man if he had ignored people's situations and worked for money alone. Yet he cared enough to put aside fees if he felt people could not pay and threw himself into helping disadvantaged and disabled people, especially children. He greatest desire was for people to be out of pain and able to function and reach their potential, and he spent long hours trying to achieve this.

We are sure that if he knew that so many were practicing "Bowen", and that his work had been written up in dozens of magazines and professional journals as well as a book, he would be amazed, but happy that his struggle had produced recognition. If he knew that his work had reached overseas he would hardly believe it.

The following is an anonymously attributed piece of writing he had on his wall. He lived by these words.

I expect to pass through this world but once
Any good thing therefore that I can do,
Or any kindness I can show to any fellow creature,
Let me do it now.
Let me not defer or neglect it,
For I shall not pass this way again.

We thank Julian and Louise for giving us this opportunity to say "hello". Every success.

Pam Trigg and Heather Edmonds, nee Bowen. Melbourne, Australia.

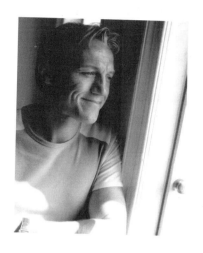

Foreword

I first came across The Bowen Technique whilst at a crucial stage of training for the 1998 London Marathon. With about two months to go before a race I was passionately looking forward to running, disaster struck. Suddenly under the weight of an unfamiliar amount of miles pounding around Hampstead Heath, an old twisted pelvis injury reared its head. After trying to run through and compensate for it I found myself in a crumpled mess with severe sciatic pain, feeling certain that my chances of making the race were extremely low to say the least.

Hardly able to walk I entered a local health clinic willing to try anything just to relieve me of my agony. By chance the little known Bowen Technique was all they had to offer (given by one Julian Baker) so I decided to have a go. One hour later I was astonished to find that the pain had all but gone, I could walk straight and furthermore running the marathon wasn't out of the question. I was especially perplexed by this apparent miracle as Julian had spent most of the session either sitting yards away on a chair or out of the room completely.

Two months later after further treatments my dream came true and I completed the race in a time I couldn't have hoped for even before the injury. Since then whenever I've had any back or neck problems, Bowen has always successfully put an end to them as well as aligning my body and increasing my energy. So I can't recommend it highly enough.

Whatever this mysterious method is, it must be learnt by more people because it really does make a difference to lives.

Star of Soldier, Soldier and Badger.

Introduction

When Tom Bowen died in 1982, he could little have imagined that in the space of the next 18 years, his name and his methods of bodywork would travel the world, giving immense relief from suffering, as well as some controversy....

Indeed even the title of this book, The Bowen Technique, is somewhat of a contradiction as Tom Bowen himself never referred to his methods as Bowen, preferring instead to call himself an osteopath, until registration of the term made this untenable due to his lack of qualifications.

Today there are many versions of Tom Bowen's work in the public domain, in dozens of countries around the world. Some use the name of Tom Bowen in their title and others draw on principles from Bowen's work but use more convoluted names. Whatever the name, one thing we can be sure of is that Bowen's work was not complete at his death and that his basic belief was that of the body's innate ability for self-recovery. He knew that if the body is given the right information and the right environment, there is little that it cannot heal itself of.

A simple principle perhaps, but one that is easily forgotten in the interventionist world of modern medicine and a principle that we will increasingly have to turn to in order to address the increasing numbers of health problems that, in spite of the extended use of drugs, we are experiencing. It is only now that we are beginning to see the wisdom in an ancient approach such as Tom Bowen's. From this humble man we can see a way of thinking which can be adapted by any modality or therapeutic discipline in order to radically change the focus from the therapist to the client.

It was Hippocrates who stated:

"The body heals itself; the physician is only nature's assistant."

With the reliance on drug-based medicine this is an ideal that has little appeal.

My purpose in writing this book is to introduce the principles of the technique as well as to define what it is that we try to achieve when using The Bowen Technique. Although I have used certain exercises to highlight some approaches to the technique, any book such as this has to state that it is not a teach-yourself Bowen book. As a teacher of The Bowen Technique, I spend many hours in classes and remain firmly convinced that only a hands-on method is possible when passing on a therapy such as Bowen. If you have already learned the technique or are thinking of attending a course, or simply want more information, then this book will open these areas up.

The Bowen Technique in Europe would not be where it is today without the dedication and extraordinary work of my wife and business partner Louise Atwill. She has managed the business side of our lives as well as raise our two children Cara and Piers, with clarity, strength and for most of the time remarkable and sorely tested patience. Louise, I thank you from the bottom of my heart.

Chapter 1
History of The Bowen Technique

Tom Bowen 1916 – 1982

The story of Tom Bowen is a remarkable one, even more so for knowing that in spite of being one of the busiest and most effective therapists of his generation, he had no formal training or qualifications in any therapeutic background.

His parents were originally from Wolverhampton and emigrated to Australia in the early 1900's, settling in Brunswick, Victoria. His was a working-class family, and Tom left school at the age of 14, taking various labouring jobs including milk carter and general hand at a woollen mill. He then went in to the building trade where he took up his father's trade of carpenter, working as a general hand at Geelong cement works.

Tom was married in the early days of World War Two to Jessie and they lived with Tom's parents in Geelong, Victoria. They were both keen Salvationists and Tom Bowen ran a Salvation Army Boy's Club which was hugely popular, where he would coach youngsters in various sports especially swimming, which was a favourite.

It was while he was working at the cement works that he started to treat people after work, coming home to wash and eat before commencing clinics that would often go well into the night. With encouragement from friends Rene and Stan Horwood, in whose house he operated his clinic, he eventually started to work full-time out of a rented house in Geelong.

Having no therapeutic background, Bowen was under no restrictions about how he should run his clinic and appointments were vague to the point of non-existent. Patients phoning for an appointment would be told to come either in the morning or afternoon. When they arrived, they were invited to take a number from a board and wait. As the clinics were only two hours long, and Bowen worked at a rate of something like fourteen patients per hour, the wait would rarely be a long one.

Talk was minimal in Bowen's clinic; patients were told not to see any other therapist and that, "If I don't get you in two (sessions) go away and save your money." Both points were good advice as Bowen was able to 'see' whether clients had indeed been treated by another therapist. In addition, patients rarely came more than twice as Bowen did not believe in extended therapy.

Another reason for minimising the chat was that Tom Bowen was profoundly deaf and wore two hearing aids, often using a method of clicking his fingers to signify to his assistants when he had finished what he was doing.

In addition to his deafness, Bowen had lost a leg through diabetes and walked around his clinic either using a prosthesis, or not, depending on his mood. He lost his second leg just prior to his death.

Romantic stories about how Bowen discovered his way of working have been spread around, including learning it in a Japanese prisoner of war camp, and spending time with Aboriginal elders where he was taught by them. Nice notions but sadly untrue.

According to evidence that he gave to the Osteopathy, Chiropractic and Naturopathic Committee Enquiry in 1973, he said that the only study he had undertaken was from books that he found useful and that all he had learned was self-taught.

All this gives an amazing overview to Tom Bowen but, personally, I believe misses the essence of how he was working and offers rather a narrow view of where the technique has come to. His work with another therapist, Ernie Saunders, has been mentioned as being a strong influence on Tom Bowen and it is surely his consistent exposure to numerous therapeutic approaches which gave Tom his 'seeing' ability.

It was often said of Bowen that he could take one look at an individual and 'see' what was wrong and from where the problem stemmed. In addition he only needed to do a few simple moves, allowing the body to rest for certain periods, before 'seeing' that the body had started to change. Once he recognised this, his work was done and the patient discharged, maybe to be brought back next week or maybe for good.

It was common for the patient to walk out in the same pain as when they had walked in, a situation that many therapists would find uncomfortable, and yet this offers an excellent opportunity to understand precisely Bowen's unique approach.

Tom Bowen's work was not a systematic series of moves or techniques but more a piece of music that would change according to the mood of the orchestra and the temperament of the conductor. What Bowen could 'see' was not something that could be put into words or classified in the strictest sense as a diagnosis. He just knew where there was an imbalance and he had the ability to know when that imbalance was changing. If you're pushing a car towards the cliff and it starts rolling, you don't need to stick around to know that it's going to go all the way. Similarly if the car is pointing downhill in the first place, then it's not going to take much of a shove to get it going.

Once Bowen had got the process moving, that was enough for him and he then knew that through the week, the body would take over and do the rest. He was rarely wrong.

The physical action he performed was secondary to the knowing *what* to perform, hence the refusal of the Osteopathic Council in 1982 to admit him as a member. Quite simply he wasn't an osteopath in the accepted sense of the word, namely diagnosing structural abnormalities and using recognised techniques to address specific problems. His disappointment with his rejection was great, especially as acceptance meant that his patients could have claimed their fees back from medical insurance and eased any financial pressure.

Bowen was a selfless man in many respects. A fortnightly clinic he ran for years, treated disabled people free of charge and he would regularly pay house calls to people who were unable to attend his clinic, even if it were in the middle of the night. On Sundays he would visit Geelong Prison to treat prisoners and was many times called upon by the Geelong Police to assist them, even being awarded a medal from the Victorian Police Board.

Bowen's Boys

Over the years in practice, Tom Bowen had many people who watched him work and who learned from him, but six men are considered to be the main ones with whom Bowen shared much of his understanding and who were regarded as 'Tom's boys'. One of the men, Oswald Rentsch claimed that Tom invited him to learn after a handshake at a conference, such was Bowen's ability to recognise the power of an individual's touch.

All of these men were physical therapists in some way, most of them having an osteopathic or chiropractic training and background. It was this formal training which gave them access to Bowen's clinic and helped them to compare methods, but paradoxically this may also have restricted their ability to look beyond a rigid format. Thus when each came to interpret what they saw, each fitted Bowen's work into a pattern that would match the basis of a structural approach. They looked for indications for specific procedures and created the 'structure governs function' methods as stated by the founder of modern osteopathy, Andrew Still.

So were they wrong in this approach? Not really, as these methods still offer validity as a mechanical and physical therapy and for the most part this is how it is taught and used around the world. It does however fall very short of the essence of bodywork if this is as far as it goes, especially when Bowen was said to have told them that all he was showing them was ten per cent of what he knew. It was up to them to go and find the rest.

Ossie Rentsch started teaching his interpretation of the work in 1982 after Bowen's death. He has claimed that Bowen commissioned him to document the work and on his deathbed told Rentsch to go and take it out into the world. This claim has never been independently verified, but it was certainly due to Ossie Rentsch that the work did indeed become as widespread around the world as it is today.

Unfortunately as with all things, there is dispute about who Bowen said what to and what exactly he did. Certainly Bowen's was not a Damascene conversion and Bowen picked up and applied many different ways of using his therapy over the years. Some people claim to teach Bowen's later or 'advanced' work whilst others boast of the purity of the method that they trumpet. This is all a red herring and stands in the way of the basic principles that surround both the man and his work. By reducing Bowen's approach to a series of moves, the essence of the work is greatly missed, even though these procedures are nearly always incredibly effective.

Bowen was not a Bowen therapist, in the same way that Christ was not a Christian. Each had a vision and a message and left it up to individuals how to interpret that message for the benefit of the people that they encountered in their lives. It is dogma and fundamentalism that over the years has clouded the understanding and adoption of the basic exhortation to go out and benefit others. Sadly the world of the therapy that carries Bowen's name is sometimes subject to disagreement and acrimony. Yet Tom Bowen was a living example of getting on with it and spent his time doing nothing except treating and helping people. As a result of this his name and principles live on today and it is this example which ultimately determines the spirit of his work and which transcends any division or minor disagreement.

The Modern Approach

As we move into the twenty-first century, a lot more is understood about the workings of the brain and how certain elemental patterns of behaviour can dictate a physical process. Most of the people working in the field of Bowen hold the man himself, Tom Bowen, as the beacon from which all things must flow and this, whilst understandable, is unfortunate. The man himself has passed on and there is no way for us to know in which direction his work would have gone and all that can be put forward is speculation.

In the true spirit of pioneers and discoverers, Bowen found a starting point from which he could encourage the body's own power of healing to take hold. What he actually discovered has huge implications in both the world of modern medicine and the complementary field. To keep the focus on what Bowen did or did not do is to live in the past and to condemn the infinite possibilities of Bowen's extraordinary discovery to the realms of idle speculation. Instead I see that The Bowen Technique is the bridge that can allow us to cross over into that part of science that has not yet understood how the brain and body co-ordinate the mass of information that allows human thought to combine with bodily function.

In time, I can see what the originator, Tom Bowen, could never have imagined, that his principles and techniques will be used as a frontline medical tool. Refused by the osteopathic community, it would be poetic justice for him to be honoured in such a way. It was said that Alexander Graham Bell had such a large vision for the usefulness of the telephone, that he made the wild prediction that one day each town would have at least two of these! Hands up those who own a mobile phone?

Chapter 2
Overview of The Bowen Technique

The Bowen Technique as we understand it today is a remedial therapy. As such the implication is that it provides a remedy but by itself this would be a limitation when it comes to talking about The Bowen Technique.

Remedy in the dictionary talks about cure, heal, resolve disease and from this perspective it places the emphasis on the therapist to perform. As I have already suggested, this is not the way that Bowen works but we will address this at a later stage.

In most societies it is very hard for people to achieve a clear balanced lifestyle without living in a hermetically sealed environment. Even if we eat a good healthy, well-balanced, organic diet, the chances are we will be exposed to stresses and conditions that our human bodies were not designed for, as we are subject to many elements beyond our personal   control. Air, water, soil quality and infection are all areas that will have an impact on the balance of our system. We are also affected by the way we travel, sit, eat, our recreation, etc.

Our exposure to physical, mental and emotional stress and the amount that we ask our bodies to do increases by the day. For the most part we take it for granted that we will be able to take on whatever comes at us, but when something goes wrong, we want things to happen quickly.

The fact that The Bowen Technique allows the body to do the work means that when there is a breakdown of the system, the process of readjustment can be rapid. A Bowen therapist does not make things happen, but simply allows the body to ask itself what needs to be done. When it happens, it is not only often very quick but also very long lasting.

The Bowen Technique is a 'hands-off, hands-on' treatment. The therapist used his thumbs or fingers on certain points around the body, making rolling type moves over the soft tissue – muscle, tendon, ligament – and in between each set of moves, leaves the room to allow a response to take effect. I will explain the breaks and the reason for them later as well as giving more detail on the move itself.

The moves are gentle and the client should experience little or no discomfort during a treatment, although there will be certain areas which might be tender or sensitive. In addition, the therapist exerts little in the way of physical effort and as such it is an ideal alternative to more physically-based treatments.

As a clinical tool Bowen is especially useful and highly effective when other treatments are unsuitable, especially in acute cases, or where a client is very frail, sick or infirm.

The treatment can be performed through light clothing, although this does require practise and many therapists continue to prefer working directly on the skin. The ultimate decision as to whether to remove clothes lies with the client.

How Many Treatments?

A piece of string question, but Tom Bowen was seeing most people for one or two treatments. Nowadays, a small number of treatments is also very much the norm, and a conversation with most Bowen practitioners will reveal that the average number of treatments is around three or four. Having said this, however, it is important to point out that there are many occasions where several treatments might be advisable or required. Also, with situations such as strokes, arthritis and other long-term illnesses, there will be no limit to the number of treatments that a client may receive, possibly over an extended period. There are also a good number of people who find great benefit from having 'top up' treatments, which both prevent them from becoming injured and keep them supple and relaxed.

How Does it Work?

For a long time various theories have been put forward to suggest how Bowen works, but in the absence of research and with little understanding of what the body does during a treatment, these have remained simply theories. However, studies carried out by Dr. Vilayanur S. Ramachandran, Professor of Neurosciences and Psychology at the University California, San Diego have, without using Bowen at all, given us a much clearer understanding of how information given to the body can be interpreted by the brain by examining cases of phantom pains in amputees.

The brain sends out electrical signals at a phenomenal rate. Something in the region of 6,000,000 impulses go out from the brain every second and these in turn come back to the brain in the shape of information. Imagine having thousands of telephones all ringing at once telling you what is going on and you will have some idea of the massive task that the brain has   in decoding the information, deciding what is valid and then acting on the relevant bits.

At any given time, the brain is having to adjust temperature, digestive enzymes, heart rate, fluid levels, hormone levels, immune system operations to name but a few of the millions of continuous calculations and decisions that are going on. This is, for the most part, without us even being aware of it, and all based on the information, reliable or otherwise, that is being fed to the brain.

The brain doesn't necessarily need to act on much of the information that it receives. In the same way, we in our daily lives are inundated with bits of information that we don't necessarily need. The decision to ignore or act upon information is often made based on past experience. We can spot a circular in the post and know that we do not need to open it. Our past experience gives us a reference point and from there, an opportunity to make a decision about how to handle the information that is being offered to us.

Similarly the brain has to use past experience in order to gain a reference point and make decisions. If we see an electric fire, then the experience of either being told as a child or the more direct experience of being burned in the past tells us to avoid touching the bars. A child's brain without this level of experience may well burn himself in order to learn the lesson.

In the burning, another lesson will be established. If I put my hand on a hot surface, a reflex in my spine makes me lift it away very quickly, with the pain of the burn kicking in a moment later. In a similar situation the small child will leave its hand there much longer until the actual pain kicks in. The pain itself is an example of the brain in action. Pain gives a signal to us firstly that something is wrong and secondly that we need to isolate the area in order to promote the responses that will start the healing process. In the case of a sprain for example, it might be that there is no actual physiological damage, but the trauma of the trip or stumble will send a signal to the brain, which will in turn isolate the area by creating pain, swelling and possibly bruising. The message to the body is **WARNING**. Do not use this area until we've got it sorted out.

Certain incidents however can override the immobility order. You might have a broken leg and be hobbling across a field on crutches, when you suddenly see a large bull thundering towards you. In an instant your brain has triggered your adrenals and a huge dose of adrenaline and other chemicals surge into your body, allowing you to run like hell, temporarily forgetting the pain of your broken leg.

The demonstration of the two-way system that the brain employs is given in Ramachandran's book, *'Phantoms in the Brain'*. He demonstrates the many different ways in which information is exchanged in the brain. In one example an amputee who had lost his right arm above the elbow, was experiencing significant phantom pains in the absent hand. It felt as if the hand was clenching into a fist and, unable to unclench due to it not being there, was creating a considerable discomfort. In this instance the motor cortex was sending the signal 'clench' to the hand. The hand was obviously unable to do this but was also unable to send a signal back via the parietal lobe to the primary motor cortex to say either that the action had been performed or that it was incapable of performing the requested clench.

Ramachandran's solution to this was very simple and demonstrates how easily the brain can be convinced, even if the information is in fact false. He created a box with two sections; into the left section he placed the left hand and into the right section the stump of the amputated arm. The box was divided by a mirror, which reflected the left hand and gave a mirror image. The appearance was as if there were both a left and a right hand in the box. In this way the brain 'saw' two hands moving freely and the signal was given to the brain that the right hand had unclenched.

You can re-create this kind of brain signal yourself. You will need another person to help you with this. Sit or stand with your arms outstretched, palms facing outwards and thumbs pointing downwards. Cross your arms over and place the palms of your hands together. Now interlock your fingers and move both hands into you, twisting your wrists until both thumbs are pointing away.

Without touching you, your partner points at any of your fingers, asking you to move the finger being pointed at. What you will find is that in spite of making a concerted effort to move the finger, another finger moves. Even if you find that you are moving the finger that has been pointed at, it will be with a conscious and determined effort that is not the normal experience of limb movement.

What this shows us is that the brain is very reliant on the information that is sent to it from the body and is inclined to accept the first version of events that it receives, even if the information is inaccurate.

When we make a Bowen move in a certain area, the brain asks certain questions of the body, in an attempt to establish what action it needs to take. In order to do this the brain goes for the information that it knows well. As we make a Bowen move the conversation between brain and body might go something like this:

Brain: What was that?
Body: I'm not really sure.
Brain: Okay, was it painful?
Body: No.
Brain: How about hot?
Body: No.
Brain: Were you scared?
Body: No… and so on.

The brain is continuing to look for points of reference that will establish what course of action needs to be taken. The Bowen move is so different, that such a point of reference is difficult to establish and the brain therefore decides that it needs to investigate further. It is at this point that the real work of the Bowen therapist begins and he leaves the room! With the therapist out of the room, the brain can quickly start to find out what happened when those moves were made. It goes into an Alpha brainwave state and the body relaxes almost immediately.

Bowen therapists will often tell you that it is a common occurrence to re-enter a room, only to have a client say: "It felt like your hands were still on me," or, "I felt a warmth or a tingling in my back." This indicates to us that the brain has asked the body for more information and attempts to effectively recreate what happened in order to decide on a course of action.

What Does it Treat?

Bowen itself doesn't treat anything and indeed one of the principles is that we don't treat specific conditions. The nice thing about Bowen is that there is no situation where it cannot be used safely and effectively. As well as structural or muscular problems, The Bowen Technique also has a profound effect on a whole range of organic conditions. The most common presentations are neck and back pain, shoulder restrictions (or 'frozen shoulder') and the general aches and pains with which we may all be afflicted.

In addition, Bowen can be useful for other less obvious problems such as ME, MS, hay fever, Irritable Bowel Syndrome, asthma, migraine, constipation, eczema and others. Once again, this is not a list that defines diseases that we can treat, more an example of the kind of conditions that can and do respond positively to Bowen treatments.

Healer or Helper

If you are a therapist reading this and you treat people with acute or chronic conditions, ask yourself this question. If a client came in pain, would I be happy if he walked out of my treatment room in the same amount of pain as when he walked in? For many therapists, especially those in the more physical therapies, the answer would almost certainly be no. You would do whatever you could to help that person out of pain there and then.

With The Bowen Technique, the approach is different and it is often not unusual for a client to walk out of the treatment room in much the same amount of pain as when they arrived. The reason for this is that the process of treatment is an ongoing one, the pace of which is determined by the client and not the therapist. In many therapies the will of the therapist is inflicted on the client. Perhaps a spinal adjustment is made, a herb is given or even a certain oil is used. In all these instances, it is very difficult for the body to refuse the work and a common comment from clients is that with certain forms of therapy, 'it goes back out again'.

With The Bowen Technique this tends to happen much less. After a treatment, a client will sometimes report feeling very tired, stiff or even unwell for several days. Sometimes 'flu' type symptoms will appear, forcing the client to go to bed for a day or two. All these are quite normal and are a sign that the brain is pushing the body to a place where it can work with the new information it has been given and set about a course of action. If you have flu, the chances are you'll go to bed and, once there, will sleep. Sleep being the ideal healing place for the body, it can work a lot faster than when you're up and running around.

Serendipity

Another variant that we often find with Bowen is what we call the serendipity effect – pleasant surprises or discoveries. A commonly reported phenomenon is one where the client returns for a second treatment reporting that yes his back, shoulder or neck is better, but that his hay fever has also cleared up, or that he hasn't had stomach pains this week.

It might well be that these other symptoms were not even mentioned during the initial consultation, as the overriding consideration had been the pain in the back, neck etc. With the information that the brain was given in the treatment, it set up a series of priorities which recognised imbalances and corrected them.

This illustrates that it is not the Bowen therapist who is doing the work or even the therapy itself but these are merely the catalysts in the process of assisting nature to do its own amazing work. The Bowen Technique acts as a bridge, a facilitator in the process of healing and recovery. This is uncommon in these days of interventionist medicine. Drugs and surgery often take over, not looking at the causes of disease or injury but only at the symptoms. An individual with knee pain having a series of investigations might only have his knee examined, even going as far as having surgery. It is likely that no-one will question whether he has any other issues, such as back, pelvic, hamstring or even bowel problems. In terms of neurological logic, a broad approach has a very scientific validity and yet is rare within modern medicine.

Things We Do Not Do

It follows that if we, as therapists, are not there to physically make people better and if we can see that the body will make adjustments to areas that we have not specifically addressed, then we have to look at our responsibilities in the role of advisor or therapist. Within the field of Bowen there are four specific things that we do not do. It is my belief that this is the manner in which most if not all complementary therapies should set their limits.

1) We Do Not Diagnose

One of the major criticisms of The Bowen Technique from people such as osteopaths, chiropractors and chartered physiotherapists, is that we do not teach (in fact we actually discourage), diagnosis in any specific manner. For some people this is seen as very limiting, but from another perspective it actually can have the opposite effect. Diagnosis by and large can be a hit and miss affair. Unless the symptoms are obvious and the experience of the therapist extensive, the process of diagnosis can end up being little more than an inspired guess.

The Bowen Technique always made it clear that any treatment is not a substitute for medical treatment. We are not doctors and don't set ourselves up as such. However what we recognise is that many people rely heavily on a diagnosis in the absence of any form of effective treatment. A good example of this is fibromyalgia. An internet search reveals dozens of pages relating to this condition. The symptoms are hugely varied and include acute joint and muscle pain, fatigue, headaches and dizziness. Run a search for ME and you'll come up with a lot of symptoms that are very similar. While no-one is suggesting for a moment that these conditions are not either serious or very distressing, it's worth pointing out that fibromyalgia actually means 'muscle or fibre pain'. It can be seen, therefore, that the diagnosis of many conditions doesn't necessarily help in the treatment or combating of the disease itself, but creates a circle of jargon that isn't always helpful.

Sometimes the client will report arthritis or rheumatism, based on the opinion of a relative, neighbour, friend or magazine article, without having had the benefit of a qualified medical opinion. Again, many clients come having seen many doctors or consultants all with differing views about what their problem may or may not be. As a result, the treatment will vary according to the opinion. Someone here has to be wrong and when that happens, the person who suffers is the patient.

Where a client comes to me asking me to give them a name for their condition I happily oblige and call it Gladys or Cynthia. Flippant, maybe, but my point is to say that firstly I am not qualified to tell them or to even venture an opinion and that secondly the actual disease itself is not foremost in my mind when talking or working with them. This brings us on to the next Bowen 'no-go' area.

2) We Do Not Treat Specific Conditions

The law in the United Kingdom is fairly generous as far as complementary therapy goes. Unlike virtually all other European countries, there are few restrictions or licensing requirements placed upon those wishing to practice the 'healing arts'. Some may say that the system is too slack and it may well be that things will change in the future, but at the time of writing, there are only a few things that we cannot treat as complementary practitioners.

AIDS and certain sexually transmitted diseases are the basic conditions that any therapist cannot treat. The wording here is very specific and clear. It says that it is illegal to treat these diseases. What it doesn't say however, is that it is illegal to treat people with any of the above mentioned diseases.

As a result I take this to the extreme, saying that as a complementary and alternative medicine profession, we should not treat any specific conditions at any time. This fits in well with the lack of diagnosis and creates a firm foundation for practice.

A client coming to me with cancer may well have a million and one problems, ranging from the cancer itself and reactions to treatments such as chemotherapy, to emotional stresses with family having to deal with their illness. The list can be exhaustive and what I want to find out, if I can, is a broader picture which gives me a point of reference that I can work with in order to best help my client.

I am not there to take away their cancer or even to suggest I can. The same applies to any condition that presents itself. The client sitting in front of you might have a textbook case of arthritis, but understanding subacromial and scapulothoracic articulations won't necessarily help you to find out that what she wants to do is to be able to put her grandchild on the swing in the park without pain. Having said this, a good foundation and understanding of anatomy and physiology is an essential part of being a confident and able practitioner.

At the same time a Bowen therapist should not attempt in any way to undermine the due medical process. It is too easy to label complementary therapies as alternative, and whilst there are definite advantages to following a more holistic approach, progress towards a more integrated health care system can only come about if the responsibility for clinical control is clearly defined.

The other point to remember, as I have already said, is that many changes can take place during a course of Bowen treatments and if we are too specific then we miss the opportunity to recognise significant serendipitous change.

As Patch Adams says in his book '*Gesundheit!*', treat the disease, some you win some you lose. Treat the patient and you win every time. Mind you he dresses as a clown and carries around a rubber fish making people crease with laughter, so he's hardly what one might call orthodox!

The late John Diamond often criticised Complementary and Alternative Medicine (CAM) for its inability to cure and yet it is this obsession with cure that can paradoxically prevent finding out where the condition comes from.

3) We Do Not Prescribe or Alter Medication

This is of course unless qualified to do so, but does include supplements, herbs and homoeopathic preparations. The reasons here are fairly obvious, but once again it comes down to clinical control, which overall is not something that I either aspire to or even believe to be necessary.

The therapist should also be careful about questioning or criticising the prescription of the original practitioner. I advise therapists that if, from experience, research, knowledge or simple gut feeling, they feel that a substance is having a detrimental effect on the client, they should advise the client to return to their GP for a re-appraisal of their original treatment or prescription. There is a difference however between prescribing or altering medication and encouraging the client to take an active role in their treatment, including asking for information about the prescribed drugs. Too often we see clients taking a combination of drugs which create a negative effect on their overall health.

From this perspective it can be very important to take a full view of the client's medication. There are several reasons for this. Firstly we need to be sure that the medication is not causing a physical reaction and thus being the reason for the client seeking treatment. Interactive drugs, where an undesirable combination of drugs is being taken, can also cause complications and although incidences of these presentations are increasingly rare, a good drugs guide is an indispensable aid to any therapist.

Another good reason for taking a drug history is that it can often give the therapist an idea about the problems that are being presented. We sometimes see clients who might be coming with a back pain, but give a list of prescribed medication that indicates a much more detailed set of circumstances. I will generally ask a client in advance to bring a list of their medication with them to avoid any forgetfulness.

Finally we need to be aware of any changes in the system as a result of the treatment. In the past it has happened that the body has changed the way it operates and as a result starts to regulate the systems normally. If medication is being given to make this happen, then reactions can occur. The most common case is diabetics who are insulin dependent. It is important with these clients that they keep a close eye on their blood sugar levels, as it has been known for Bowen to reactivate the body to produce more insulin and at least one case of hospitalisation has occurred as a result. Other conditions being regulated by medication such as high blood pressure, thyroid imbalance or fluid retention might also be affected by treatment and therefore require a re-assessment of medication.

4) We Do Not Make Claims

The final aspect of 'no-nos' is that of making claims regarding the outcome of treatment. There are never any guarantees in this world and when it comes to therapy, then it is even more important to realise this. Although we see The Bowen Technique as a very successful treatment, there are many situations and reasons why a treatment might not work.

It is impossible to ever predict this and so any client may or may not respond. There are perhaps reasons why the treatment is not succeeding and these will be dealt with in another section, but for whatever reason there are times when it just doesn't work.

To this end it is essential to avoid making any claims or predictions of outcome. It may well be that pretty much ninety per cent of all the people I see report a resolution or positive change to their problem, but that still leaves the ten per cent, some of whom naturally are disappointed. I am frequently disappointed when I see uses of the word cure or claims from 'healers' that they can rid people of illnesses or diseases. Possibly they can, but just as possibly they might not and that's when people are given false hopes that someone can take away their illness or pain.

The Power of the Mind?

People sometimes ask whether it is necessary to 'believe' that Bowen will help and whether it will have a lesser effect if the client doesn't believe that what they are undertaking is going to do them any good. This is a difficult question and the answer is both a yes and a no.

I have seen people who believe so firmly that what I will do is going to work, that even if it doesn't they still feel much better. One lady convinced herself that she had much more movement through her shoulder, when in fact it had remained exactly the same for a long time. She felt better in herself and much more cheerful and therefore one could say that the outcome was quite satisfactory. Outcomes after all are for the client not the therapist, a point that is very easily missed by those with egos that need to be massaged.

Conversely I have had many sceptics who have sat in front of me swearing blind that they think I'm a crackpot and that they don't believe a word of what I'm saying. These people need to be wised up a bit before we continue and I am more than happy to give them the option of leaving. After all they're not there for my benefit and if they truly don't think that it's going to be of any use, then they might as well forget it. To date no-one has left, leaving me with the feeling that perhaps they want to believe or at least are prepared to show a chink in their credibility factor. Pretty much all of these have been men and most if not all of them have had a one hundred per cent recovery. In more than one case however, they have denied that either there has been any recovery (in spite of playing tennis for the first time in four years) or that there wasn't much of a problem in the first place. This again in spite of extensive notes which demonstrate something very different.

I don't think that an overwhelming belief is necessary for recovery, and yet conversely a totally accepting mind is not always useful either. When I had my first Bowen treatment whilst living in Australia, I was used to a very heavy touch that had been applied during treatments of something called 'Re-balancing'. This consisted of deep tissue manipulation not unlike Rolfing or Heller work. It was for the most part exceedingly challenging and painful and resulted in a lot of yelling during the treatment. From this I formed the impression that this was how therapy was supposed to be. If it didn't hurt it wasn't going to help, 'no pain no gain'. My opinion of soft tissue treatments was therefore very harsh and based on a set of truisms that applied only to my own personal experiences.

My initial view of Bowen was that it was rubbish and could offer me nothing. Despite being in acute pain from a neck problem which had been bothering me off and on for years, I was very resistant to the light moves that the therapist was making. In addition she kept on leaving the room and had not warned me in advance that this is what would happen.

By the end of the treatment a couple of things were happening. Firstly I had virtually run out of patience. The endless trips out of the room were bad enough, but when she was actually present, she seemed to do nothing. Secondly, at the end of the session I was in the same amount of pain as when I had walked in and to be then asked to return the following week seemed to be an outrage. On top of that she charged me $30 and I had the feeling I had been truly 'done'. I had no intention of going back the second week and left feeling cheated and still sore. The next day however I had to face up to the annoying reality that my neck pain was in fact eighty per cent improved. By that evening it had virtually gone completely and by three days following the treatment, the pain and restriction were a distant memory.

Naturally enough this led me on to learning the technique but ensured that I never worried if a client didn't believe it would 'work'.

All in What Mind?

Part of the discussion about how much the mind controls the body should not be confused with the concept of mind so please forgive me if I give a brief explanation of the difference. You can eat the brain but you can't eat the mind. The brain is a piece of functional tissue that can be weighed, dissected, looked at, smelt and felt. With the mind you can do none of these and yet we attribute a huge amount of power and influence to the mind.

The analogy of brain, body and mind relationship is that of a computer. The keyboard, screen, mouse and box that hold it all together are our body. The hard disk is the brain that stores all the information and enables all the bits to come together and work as one. The computer can become damaged and when both the hardware and software are also affected, it doesn't work properly.

The mind is the software that gets imprinted on to the hard disk. It can be wiped off, changed, corrupted and can also be transferred from one worn out bit of hardware to another. It deals with all thoughts and considerations and is affected by things such as belief, habit, faith, and so on. Essentially all three need to exist in order for a human to function, but even though they exist separately they are all seriously affected by each other.

Attitudes are a good example of a state of mind. They can change radically over quite short periods of time according to different sets of circumstances. When you're sixteen the world can seem a relatively unfair place. You consider yourself to be an adult, restricted in your ability to do the things you want by people older than yourself who really haven't got a clue how it all really should be. This is an example of mind at work. Within the field of therapy there are attitudes that can have an overriding effect on the outcome of treatment and can cancel out any effect that the brain and body might decide is beneficial. There are many reasons why this might happen and we will cover some of these later.

Mind is a subject that comes up quite often for therapists looking for reasons as to why a technique might work (or not). For the medical profession the phrase 'all in the mind' is one used readily when referring to complementary medicine or diseases that don't fit into the conventional view. It's convenient as it means that there is no real need to take things like Bowen very seriously. Research into this area is time consuming and generally expensive as we found out when conducting a research programme ourselves. This is covered under the research chapter.

Beds or Tables

Bowen had a slightly unorthodox approach to treatment and although there are certain elements that would not be helpful to mimic, other factors are worth a look. One of these was the surroundings he worked in. It's worth remembering that as Bowen had no formal training he therefore had no sense of right or wrong in regard to clinical practice and subsequently set his own standards of practice and as already mentioned his approach to the running of his clinic was somewhat unorthodox by today's standards.

This also extended to his use of soft single beds. Although he was very keen on these to work on, when he saw electric tables that raised up and down, he immediately bought two. From my own perspective I still prefer a bed to work on wherever possible and the reason for this is simply what the brain says when it sees a bed.

In our own homes, the place that we would generally go to in order to get some peace and quiet would be the bedroom. The bed is conducive to sleep which hopefully for most people is a pleasant and relaxing experience. A therapy table can these days be made to extremes as far as width, comfort, softness etc., but it does still remain a therapy table.

The environment for treatment can be a good part of how the client feels before, during and after their session and a bed can contribute greatly to this experience. In my treatment room I have a single bed that is raised to the height of a low massage couch. It is covered with a sheet, with a towel on top and a piece of couch paper on top of that.

To the eye it appears to be a therapy table, albeit a low one. When the client lies down they are often surprised to find that it is indeed soft and very comfortable. Immediately the brain switches from the thought 'therapy table' and the equation of therapy to the pain or discomfort that they are in, to 'bed, relax, sleep'.

I realise that for some people the idea of a bed in a room is one that they might find disturbing bringing as it might some suggestions of improper conduct. If in doubt don't do it, but all I can say is that from experience it is very effective.

One practitioner told me: "I was getting what I considered to be excellent results and as I was doing Bowen more and more, decided to switch over to using a bed that I had raised. I couldn't really see how my results could possibly improve, but it was quite remarkable. People just relaxed immediately and the changes both during and after the session were quite profound."

The other point about beds is that they do not have a face hole. Again from a personal perspective I find this no bad thing as I have never found face holes to be particularly comfortable. If they were, surely we would find divan beds with them in as a feature, with a dribble bucket underneath, perhaps?

From an anatomical view, the use of a face hole is there so that work can be done on the neck whilst the client is prone. This applies mainly to massage and as we do not work on the neck with the client prone, the need for the face hole is removed. The forehead also is pushed backwards under pressure when in a face hole and this in turn puts the thoracic area into tension. Client comfort is, however, paramount and if we find that there is a neck restriction and that lying prone is uncomfortable, then we can put a pillow or cushion under the chest which will ease any discomfort and allow the client to lie in a prone position pain free.

As with anything we discuss around Bowen or in this book, there is a need to be adaptable and flexible and nothing here is cast in stone. If you can't work on a bed, work on a table, and if that isn't available, work on a chair or the floor. Doing something, however inconvenient, is generally better than doing nothing because it's too much bother.

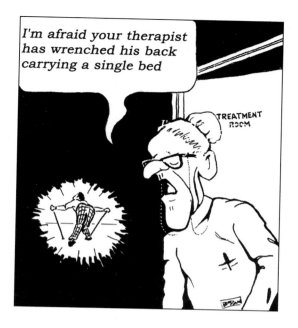

Rooms

The room that you use for treatment should overall be one that you would find relaxing or pleasant to be in. Too often therapists mistake the need to be professional with the need to be clinical, ending up with rooms that are more like hospital mortuaries than places of healing and relaxation. For relaxation is the key here. It has long been recognised by the medical establishment that the majority of presentations to GP's are illnesses related to or exacerbated by stress. It follows from this that the antidote to stress is relaxation and this is something that many people are unable to achieve and indeed misunderstand. To be relaxed doesn't mean to fall asleep, as sleep in itself can be a way of blocking stressful situations. Relaxation is being able to be fully involved in a situation without getting stressed in the first place. In other words seeing things clearly and with a balanced and calm view. A relaxed person would not be all floppy and dozy, but would be alert both physically and mentally, able to make decisions and take action without being subject to palpitations, panic attacks, headaches or other physical or mental symptoms.

During a treatment, a client should feel that there are no distractions that are going to detract from them being the focus. Ideally the room should be quiet, warmer than average without being stuffy, of a gentle colour, uncluttered and without external noise. There should be no telephones ringing and any computers or other such equipment should be turned off. I always give the client the choice of having music or having a quiet time and most people choose the latter.

It's very rare that people have a chance to simply lie quietly without the stimulus of music, chatter, telephones and such like and it is often assumed by therapists that a relaxation tape is relaxing to everyone. When people do choose music, I ask them if they have any preference and if not try to choose something as neutral as possible. New age music can often be all bells and whale songs and often quite annoying. I generally choose a piece of gentle piano music but nothing too strident and check whether this is pleasing to the client.

Reactions

It is not uncommon for people to have reactions from The Bowen Technique and it can be for this reason that people will seek other therapies. Handling reactions is a very important part of treatment and can make the difference between success and failure.

When we offer treatment, there is no way that we can predict the outcome. What we are hoping for is change and this change can come in many different ways. The obvious change is that of improvement but there are many instances where the condition worsens before any improvement is seen. The phrase 'healing crisis' is often used in these situations but I prefer to use the term, 'healing process', as it is part of the process that the client is undergoing. Crisis is an implicitly negative word, although it is worth remembering that in Chinese, crisis and opportunity are the same word.

Common reactions can be those of extreme fatigue, stiffness or soreness in the area of concern, headaches or flu-like symptoms. For most people however there is nothing more than a little tiredness or stiffness and in a lot of cases there are no reactions at all.

Headaches are a common reaction to treatment and a good clue as to whether enough water is being taken in. In some cases a headache will start even before the treatment has finished. Other situations can arise where the current symptoms are exacerbated and even increased in intensity. Old problems might re-emerge with aches and pains that have not been around for years, suddenly coming back with a vengeance. Once again it is important to view any reactions like this within the context of acceptable change.

Reactions like outcomes are difficult to predict, but the therapist who sees strong reactions on a regular basis should take a good look at whether they themselves are implicated in these, as it could well be that too much work is being done.

Although unpredictable, positive and patient support is vital when handling the client who is having a strong reaction. I always advise that the therapist should not warn the client that reactions are a possibility. The reasons for this are mainly to avoid 'setting the client up' for a reaction that they might otherwise not have had. In most cases however it isn't necessary as there simply won't be any reaction at all. I therefore leave the option for the client to phone if they have any problems.

Anyone who is having a reaction and is worried by it will generally call fairly quickly after the treatment and when this happens we need firstly to establish confidence in the process and be positive. "I'm feeling terrible," says the client; "Great," says the therapist, thereby ensuring a punch on the nose at the next visit. While a positive response to a client's reaction is good, a balance needs to be achieved and the best way around this is gentle reassurance.

In some cases a client might ask: "What did you do to me?" It's an ideal chance to answer the question with a question and be literal about it. "Okay what did I do?" From this view what I did was actually very little, putting in gentle, painless moves, leaving the room for two minutes at a time and ending the session with the client feeling relaxed. I didn't massage deeply or apply deep or prolonged pressure. I didn't adjust bones or make hard sharp adjusting type movements. When the client compares what has been done to how they are feeling, they can often see that there is an inequality that demonstrates that something quite profound is going on.

If the reactions persist, then it might be that a re-injury has occurred or that other factors need to be taken into account. Remember that any reaction is an indication that the treatment is prompting movement and that this is an excellent sign.

"I can't come back and have that again, it made me feel too ill." It's a comment that some Bowen therapists have had from people who have had reactions, but one that must be dealt with. Once again it's down to the process and it's important that the client understands this. I use the analogy of the person who decides to have their lounge room and dining room knocked into one. Having got two or three quotes, the selected builders arrive one morning armed with sledgehammers and a skip outside the front door. As the customer goes off to work several hefty builders are giving his living room wall what for. That evening he comes home from work to find what? Of course the builders have finished, cleaned up, vacuumed the room and left, leaving behind a friendly note and a bunch of flowers. The lounge room has now become a lounge diner, all the plaster is dry and both rooms have been freshly decorated in the most exquisite of colours. Oh, and your lottery numbers came up too!

In reality of course the customer returns home to find a mess. The wall in his lounge room has a gaping hole, half the ceiling is hanging down and the whole house is covered in a fine layer of dust. In the kitchen there are eight chip wrappers and seventeen dirty coffee mugs, two of which are chipped. However trying this might be, it is unlikely that the customer will tell the builders that the whole process is too messy and confrontational and that they should stop. After all, if he did, then he would be left with a mess that he would be unable to fix. Instead he realises that the process of getting his lounge diner will entail mess and change and so keeps his eye on where he will be, rather than where he is. In the same way we can see that clients can often have unrealistic expectations regarding the outcome of treatment. It might be that they want a resolution, but that the change that might be involved to get there is simply too confronting. As therapists we also need to be sensitive to this and avoid over-working.

Aftercare

As well as explaining the importance of not mixing treatment, there are things that we need to outline regarding what the client can expect and what they must do. We can sum up the bulk of the aftercare quite simply, by calling them the 3 W's. Water, Walk and Week.

Water

Water is probably one of the most underrated and underused medicines of our time. For Bowen therapists it's one of the key tools in the care of clients. Our bodies are made up primarily of water and yet few people drink much water, with many people confessing to neither drinking nor liking water. Water is responsible for the smooth operation of most of our body systems including cell production, lymphatic movement, digestion, toxin removal and so on. Plasma, the straw-coloured liquid that is found in blood and lymph, constitutes about 55% of blood and is 90% water and is key in the movement of water between blood and body tissue. In his book, 'Your Body's Many Cries For Water', Dr. F. Batmanghelidj has re-written the textbooks on the approach to the use of water in medicine and the sub-heading for his book is, 'You are not sick, you are thirsty'.

In his book, Dr. Batmanghelidj refers to the point that many medical practitioners are unaware of the many chemical roles of water in the body.

"Because dehydration eventually causes the loss of some functions, the various sophisticated signals given by the operators of the body's water rationing programme during severe and lasting dehydration have been translated as indicators of unknown disease conditions of the body. This is the most basic mistake that has deviated clinical medicine."

A key question for Bowen therapists to ask will be, "Do you drink much water?" For most people the answer is nearly always no and this in turn can create problems. In many cases, the problems that the client is complaining of are caused, or can be resolved by simply increasing the intake of water. Bowel and digestive problems are the major ones, but Dr. Batmanghelidj refers to asthma and allergies, high blood cholesterol, hiatus hernia and hypertension as all being conditions that are exacerbated by lack of water and therefore can be assisted by the intake of water.

The general thought that occurs to most people when you ask them to drink water, is the vision of large glasses of water that they will have to gulp down and the subsequent increase in visits to the toilet. For the most part this isn't the most effective way to increase health through drinking water, as most of the re-hydrating benefits will be lost through urination. Instead, the recommendation is to drink small amounts frequently. The aim is for the average person to drink at least two litres of water a day, increasing this amount in hot weather or when exercising. By drinking 100ml every 20 minutes or so, this target can be easily reached and most people will not experience much in the way of an increase in urination.

After a Bowen treatment, the body will use water reserves to start the process of elimination of toxins and other dysfunctional debris and water is therefore an important element for avoiding and controlling reactions to treatment. This isn't about to turn into a treatise on the benefits of water – there are other excellent books that can do that. Neither will I go into the debate regarding the drinking of mineral water over tap water, suffice to say that I regard the drinking of any water as beneficial and for many people the purchasing of expensive bottled water is not an option.

There is a big difference between water and other fluids, and tea and coffee do not count as water intake. Neither for that matter do herbal teas, juices or cordials. Once again however, I will refer you to other weightier tomes for greater detail. Encouraging clients to drink water is incredibly beneficial and I am convinced that the drug bill for the UK alone would plummet if people were encouraged simply to drink more water.

Walk

As well as water for lymph production, the lymphatic system relies on contraction of skeletal muscle to move lymph around the body, although there is a suggestion that lymph nodes themselves may have some sort of pumping action that assists this process. We all know the benefit of exercise to increase the heart rate and the huge number of advantages that come about with a regular programme of exercise. For many people however, exercise equates to putting on shorts and going to the gym and yet simply walking, even gently, can have an inordinate effect on the body.

After treatment, movement is terribly important and for this reason we ask that a client, on the day of a treatment, avoid sitting down for more than half an hour at a time. This is in order to keep the body systems active and encourage removal of debris and toxins. In conjunction with the drinking of water, this will help the process of system change and go some way towards preventing excessive reactions. The actions of standing and walking also go some way towards reminding the body that it has undergone treatment and restart the process almost every time. This extends to clients who have travelled some distance or have to drive a long way on the day of treatment. If they are going to be in the car for longer than half an hour, they should pull over and walk around the car, before getting back in and driving on. It may sound trivial, but the difference it has made in the past between success and otherwise is quite remarkable.

Even after the day of treatment, I recommend that clients set a timer to ensure that they are not sitting at their desk or on the sofa for extended periods of time.

Week

The optimum time for the second treatment is five to ten days after the first one, with seven being preferable. One of the features of Bowen is that we do not treat every day, except in exceptional circumstances, in order to allow the body to implement the changes in its own time. Once again it is important to remember that it is not the therapist who is doing the work, but the body, and for this to be effective, it needs to have some time to react. The key word here is 'repair', and for this to happen, the therapist needs to back off. I once visited a sports therapist who was working with a professional football team. While I was there he was working on a player who had strained his hamstring. I asked him how he would be treating the player and how often. He replied that after some ice to the area, he would then proceed over the next few days to treat it every day, using various methods of treatment including massage, ultra sound and a heat lamp. The question that I wanted to ask was, "When did the player's own body have a chance to jump in and have a go?"

The body is the healer and however tempting it might be, we have to resist the desire to keep pushing and pushing to get a result. Time and trust are two key elements in working with the principles of The Bowen Technique and once a therapist can understand these, then truly wonderful things will happen. Allowing the body to undertake its own repair, means that when the work is done it will generally stay done and not need to be constantly worked on.

One of my constant frustrations is the sight of professional athletes, soccer players in particular, who keep getting re-injured unnecessarily. The reason for this continuing state of affairs is that the original injuries have never been fully treated and given a chance to repair, giving rise to injury on injury and in some cases cutting short the careers of otherwise healthy and talented players. I have no doubts that Bowen can revolutionise sport in general and soccer in particular, once certain hardened and old-fashioned attitudes change and the role of the individual in their own healing is   recognised. As with any rule however there are some exceptions to the seven-day approach.

Re-injury

This is one of those vast areas where pretty much the most minor of incidences could be considered to constitute a re-injury, but for the most part we are talking about the obvious. A more detailed explanation of the various levels of re-injury will come later. In this instance an example would be that of the footballer whom we have treated on one day and who two days later gets kicked, or falls and experiences the same pain again. In addition he might also have injured another area but, in either case, we would ask him to come back before his scheduled second treatment. This doesn't just apply to sports people, but to any individual.

Pregnancy

A pregnant woman can experience lots of problems, and is naturally facilitating a process of rapid and remarkable change. From one day to the next there will be changes and the baby inside her is growing at a phenomenal rate. As a result, we can work with this and, if necessary, treat her every day. Bowen is also an incredibly useful tool during labour, with many midwives using it as an intrinsic part of their work.

Brain Damage

In this case we are talking in particular about situations such as strokes, cerebral palsy etc., and once again we can treat more than once a week, but usually not more than twice. The reasoning behind this is that the information that we are asking the brain to absorb is not being delivered effectively. Once again it is important to remember that we are not treating the condition, but the person themselves and so must resist simply looking for results that put too much emphasis on resolution or physical outcomes.

With these conditions we are going to be working with the client on a long-term basis and three or four treatments will provide little change.

Terminal Illness

Where we are working with a terminally-ill client, the parameters of treatment change completely and in many ways the whole approach of working with the person and not the disease becomes clearer. We are all going to die and yet for most people this is not something that they consider from one day to the next. I think that this is a sad state of affairs. What has happened is that death and dying have become a scary, secretive thing that is removed and sanitised in order to give some sort of misplaced protection from a distasteful subject. To work with someone who is dying gives an amazing opportunity for the therapist to focus on the individual and be with them in each moment. At the same time it can offer a tremendous opportunity to understand the nature of our own mortality. I sincerely hope that one day we will have midwives for the dying, helping people to die and plan for their own deaths with compassion and positivity. When this happens I am sure that tools such as Bowen will have a major part to play. If you find yourself in this situation however, all the rules go out of the window and your task is simply to apply whatever skill or knowledge you have in order to best help the person you are with. Mixing therapies is not only allowed here, but is actively encouraged. Remember that death is an outcome just like any other. The negativity or otherwise of it is a state of mind.

Chapter 3
Four Major Principles of The Bowen Technique

As we have already mentioned, there are several schools of thought about what Tom Bowen did or did not do and with the man himself no longer around to correct the more absurd claims, we have to regard what few facts we have. There remain in force about four major principles that underpin The Bowen Technique as we understand it: The Bowen Move, The Stoppers, The Breaks, Bowen – the Jealous Lover of Remedial Massage. Although these might seem to be a bit thin on the ground, there is actually a mass of information contained within them. The first principle and the one that makes The Bowen Technique instantly recognisable is:

I. The Bowen Move

The Bowen move itself is like a complete work of art and is in essence both the beginning and the end of what we refer to as The Bowen Technique. When observed it looks and indeed is, very simple. Yet the move starts as a series of events, which change the whole energetic and physical structure of the body. It allows a flow of communication between all the organs, systems, cells and extremities and, in addition, initiates a level of dialogue with the therapist. Viewed simply, it is just the movement of a bit of tissue and skin, in much the same way as a Mozart piano concerto is a jolly little tune.

After reading this book you may well have a good idea of what the technique is all about. You may even be able, having studied it carefully to imitate the nature of the move that I am trying to explain but in reality, without the feel and the experience of what the move is, this attempt will be pretty hollow.

The best way therefore to proceed from here is to try and break things down into sections that are easily digestible and the Bowen move does happen to have three distinct parts that adapt to this explanation well.

a. The Skin Slack
b. The Pressure used to move the skin slack and also to make the move
c. The Move itself

We are going to look first at (b), the Pressure, in order to better understand the differentiation between the pressure required to move the skin and that required to make the move.

(b) Eyeball Type Pressure

We refer to the pressure that we use as eyeball, but this can be actually quite misleading. If you press on to your eyeball (with your eyes closed please) then you will find that you are unable to apply much in the way of pressure before it becomes uncomfortable or before the other eyeball lands on your lap. If you have ever experienced a Bowen treatment then you will know that the therapist generally applies a degree more pressure than this. The point here is not how much pressure is used, but rather the type of pressure.

When you press your eyelid with the eyeball underneath, you are setting up a level of communication between yourself and your eyeball, with the middleman being your brain. Your fingers are judging how much pressure you can apply without hurting yourself, and your eyeball is giving you feedback about when to stop before you do hurt yourself.

In essence this is no different to how one should approach the pressure when treating a client. The therapist's fingers need to develop in order to ascertain exactly how much pressure can be applied in order to create the best effect within the comfort zone of the client.

Too much and you stand the chance of hurting someone, too little and you might not be creating the stimulus to the nerve endings which might benefit the body the most. Balance is what we are after. Initially it's a fine line and inevitably practitioners get it wrong. I have been treated by experienced teachers of the technique and have been dismayed by the heavy pressure used and subsequent pain that has occurred. On the other hand I have also been treated by therapists using a very light touch and this in turn, although effective has left me with a feeling of wanting to feel a little more. The touch that I try to describe is one whereby the client is aware of where the therapist is moving, but at all times could have more pressure applied without feeling pain. The key to Bowen is that it is very gentle. Many people are surprised and even a little put out that there is such a light pressure involved, especially sportsmen who might be used to a heavier touch with deep tissue massage or other techniques.

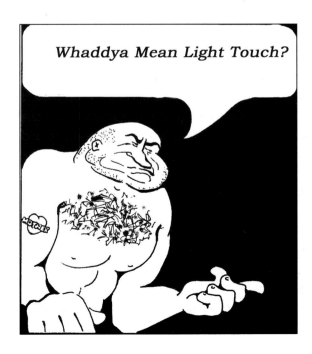

There are two types of pressure needed when performing Bowen, however, and a distinction should always be drawn. The type of pressure needed to make the move is that of eyeball type, but a much lighter pressure is used to move the skin around, which in turn allows us to access the muscle or tendon on the area we wish to work. This brings us neatly to;

(a) Skin Slack

Skin slack is the skin which both works for and against us when we are using The Bowen Technique. In order to get at a particular muscle and move over it, we need to get rid of the excess skin that sits on top of the area. When we have moved this skin away, we then use it to, in effect, 'ride' it over the muscle or tendon. We all have varying degrees of skin over our body, but one area in which we can easily demonstrate this is the back of our hand. If we put the first two fingers of our right hand on the back of our left hand, we can feel that there is an amount of skin that can be moved around. Whenever we make a Bowen move, there is never any sliding and so if we imagine that our fingers have been stuck to the back of our hand, then we know that we cannot slide anywhere.

What we can also feel is that there is a limit as to how far we can go with our fingers in any direction. If we go beyond the limit of the skin then we have to slide. At this stage we are moving the skin around without paying much attention as to how much pressure we need to use to do this. If we focus, we can see that we only need the lightest of touches, much less than the eyeball type, in order to move the skin around on the back of the hand. This is both skin slack and a demonstration of the pressure that we need to apply in order to move skin.

(c) The Move

The Bowen move is the combination of the correct amount of pressure with the removal of the skin slack. The move itself is a roll over the muscle, tendon or ligament in whatever area we are working. When we make a Bowen move it's important to remember that it isn't just that particular muscle or tendon that is being affected, but that the whole body is having to respond to each and every move that we make.

A Bowen move should not be a flick or a twang of a muscle. In the past it has been compared to the plucking of a guitar string, but this is to misunderstand the nature of what the move is intended to do. Everything has a frequency, meaning a vibration at a certain level. A way that engineers test whether a large concrete building has stress fractures is to send a vibrational frequency up the building and measure the reading that comes back. In the same way the brain is acting like a radar, that is picking up a movement or vibration in the body and is asking for more information.

The Bowen move should not be painful and although there will be times that we find tender spots, the overall treatment should not be viewed as uncomfortable.

In an attempt to describe a move that is very hard to describe, I ask the reader for patience and a level of imagination. The therapist stands on the left side of the client and positions his hands approximately 2.5cms away from the spine around the lower back on the same side that he is standing. Exactly where on the back this is doesn't matter for the moment, placement will come later. The tips of the thumbs are together and should be lightly resting on top of the large erector spinae group of muscles that support the spine. The thumbs gently draw as much skin as possible towards the therapist, applying only the pressure required to move the skin.

On the client exhaling, the therapist applies pressure to the outside – lateral – aspect of the muscle with the pads of the thumbs and then starts to slowly move the hands forward, whilst at the same time lifting the wrists. As the thumbs roll over, the muscle, which is under pressure, moves backward towards the therapist in a gentle roll which can be felt under the thumbs.

The move on the other side of the erector spinae is performed with the fingers. The index fingers of both hands start on the belly of the erector spinae, and push the skin away. As the skin moves away the fingers follow the shape of the muscle, creating a curve in the fingers. Pressure is then applied by gently pulling towards the spine. As this action is applied, the hands move medially and the fingers start to straighten, once again creating the rolling effect in the muscle that typifies The Bowen Technique move.

The way to remember this is that the skin slack is always moved in the opposite direction to the move. The movement of the muscle actually is an opposite reaction to the move that the therapist makes.

While the move itself carries a huge amount of information, the skilled therapist will be gathering information at the same time as making the move itself. Heat, cold, skin condition, tension of the muscle, general response on making the move and looking at these from the point of comparing from one side to the other. It's a lot to expect that someone will achieve all of this, but simply getting the move in a careful and controlled way is the initial goal.

The move actually varies very little when moving around the body, sometimes using the heel of the hand or on occasion the elbow. Because, however, the move will have a different effect every time, there comes a time when one is learning the move every time it is performed.

The next principle that is part of the make-up of Bowen is an interesting one that in essence is difficult to quantify and that is;

2. The Stoppers

The stoppers or blockers although implying that they stop or block, actually do the opposite, creating a sort of opening effect.

As well as being functional, the stopper moves are also remedial and are two of the most important moves in the Bowen repertoire. The lower stoppers are the first moves that are performed in any treatment and also represent one of the few hard and fast rules that are applied in advanced work. This is that they are always done first, as an assessment move, and are generally repeated before commencing with other moves or assessments.

The moves that make up the stoppers are the same as described previously for the basic move. What makes the stoppers what they are, however, is the location. The location for the lower or bottom stoppers is on the most concave point of the curving spine that we, as humans, possess. The simple reason for us having a curve in the spine is that we are the only mammals that walk upright and the curve has the effect of a shock absorber for a series of bones that would quickly crumble if the spine were straight. As with any suspension system however, there are points that are going to absorb more shock than others and it is the extremities of the curve that will get the most in the way of stress.

As a result of this, the muscular structure either side of the spine at these points will tend to be stronger, tighter, more prone to aches and pains and hold more energy. Hence the upper thoracic area and the mid to lumbar areas are, in my experience, the areas that most people will have stiffness and soreness on a regular basis.

As remedial moves, the stoppers address the tension in this area, which in turn has to have a knock on effect on the whole spine and therefore the whole body. There is more to this however than just a relaxation of the spine. When we make a medial move with our fingers or thumbs, the muscle has to react and move in the opposite direction, hence our medial move actually creates an opening effect on the erector spinae group.

The opening of the erector spinae group focuses the brain onto the region in which we are working and from that point, the work we do beneath this area has become a kind of VIP section. It's a little like rolling back a big stone to open up a cave. Once inside, your normal voice and the sounds you make become accentuated by the openness of space. In the same way, once we have put our stoppers in around the lower back, then anything we subsequently do has more volume and resonance than it did previously.

The stoppers in the upper back are, once again located at the extreme curve of the spine, this time the most convex part of the upper thoracic area. In this area we actually apply four moves instead of the two that are the lower stoppers. The reason for this is the level of energetic movement that there is around the upper thoracic and also the level of spinal cord activity. In this area the nerve endings from T5–T8 deal with the stomach, pancreas, spleen, liver, digestion and duodenum.

Once we have applied the sets of stoppers, both upper and lower, we have, in effect, cut the body into three sections. Although the main implications of this come mosty into the later more advanced work, it essentially gives us options over where we can work and the order that we can apply procedures.

A variation of stoppers is 'holding points' and these are used in various points where moves need to be diverted or re-directed. The holding points are, in effect, temporary stoppers, only being in place while the therapist has his fingers on the point and is released when the fingers are.

3. The Breaks

Another principle of Bowen is that, as well as doing very little in the way of hands on physical work, in between these sets of moves the therapist leaves the room for a short period. These breaks can initially be quite a confronting exercise, mainly for the therapist who has been trained in therapies where a strong component is to keep contact with the body at all times.

The breaks, however, are an important element of Bowen and one that should be explored. I have heard it suggested that Tom Bowen only left the room so that he could go and treat other people. If this was the case, then why didn't he just do shorter treatments? This cynical view fails to appreciate the importance of allowing what the therapist has just done to take effect. If we go back to the concept of how Bowen actually works then we see that there is a level of communication between the body and the brain. The small moves send a vibration or a physical signal to the brain, which then has to determine what has happened and decide on the course of action it will take. In order for this to happen, there need to be a few parameters in place.

Firstly there cannot be too much information going to the brain at any one time. Think of a daily thing like, for instance, a shopping trip to the supermarket. It might be that we look in the cupboards and decide that we only need a few things and don't need to write a list. By the time we get to the supermarket, our brain has undertaken literally millions of individual calculations, assessments and tasks and dealt with countless pieces of information. Even with this we can still remember some of the things we need. If you are like me, getting into the supermarket changes all of this and suddenly you are bombarded with masses of items that you don't need, coming out with half of what you wanted and a lot of what you didn't.

With Bowen it is similar and we therefore need to try and assess what the body needs, give it only the amount of information it can take, and then leave it to work out what is being asked. Tom Bowen, as we have already stated, was not a Bowen therapist as we understand the profession today and the working practices of modern practitioners would have very little resemblance to the way the man himself operated. It's worth remembering that Bowen had an innate ability to see the effects of the moves and knew when sufficient work had been done. As with anything very visual however, one needs a comparison and so leaving the room not only gave the body the chance to use the information it needed, but also gave Bowen the space to see what had changed. It also meant that he could treat someone else as well.

Why can't we stay in the room? This is a question that is regularly asked and, in some cases, we can and should stay with the client. When I first had a Bowen treatment, the therapist kept on leaving the room and had not explained to me at the outset that this is what she would be doing. The frustration that I experienced while lying there as she disappeared, not knowing why, was immense and led me to be clear in the way that I explain the process to my clients before treatment begins. As part of this I also explain the concept of leaving the room and ask if this will be okay with them. In some instances, probably about four over the years, I have had some people say that they would rather I stayed in the room with them and this, naturally, I have done.

The reason that we leave is for the client to be very much in their own space and without external or distracting stimulus. It is very rare for people in our society to take time wherein they just sit or lie, without the distraction of TV or conversation and a Bowen treatment provides an ideal opportunity to do just that. If I am asked to stay in the room then I ask the client to lie quietly and then try to sit as far away from them as possible.

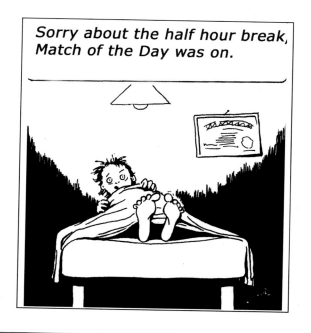

For some therapists the set up of their room means that they will be unable to step outside and, once again, in this case they should try and create some kind of screen or separation to suggest that the client is by themselves. The temptation to chat aimlessly is also a strong one when the therapist stays in the room and one that should be avoided.

Once again there are a few exceptions to the rule of leaving the room and these are based on common sense rather than any deeply held ethic. When working with children there are a couple of rules to observe and these will be covered in more detail in the section on working with children, (see page 56). However it is unwise to leave the room when working with a child. The other exceptions are those who request that you stay and very elderly people. If you get the feeling that you should stay, then stay, at least until you are happy that it is all right for you to leave.

Eventually the Bowen therapist uses the breaks as an opportunity to re-assess when coming back into the room. If things have changed then there is the chance to react to the changes and alter the treatment accordingly.

4. Bowen – The Jealous Lover of Remedial Therapy

One significant element of The Bowen Technique is the emphasis on the client not having any other form of treatment whilst undergoing Bowen. In some cases it can be quite unpopular but this is mainly from the side of therapists who feel their hands are tied.

Tom Bowen was very specific regarding this and had the ability to tell when a client had seen another therapist during the week. When it transpired that they had, he would refuse to treat them and ask them to leave. It might sound harsh, but the end result was that most people knew where they stood with him, and therefore didn't mix their treatments.

There are a number of reasons why we don't mix the treatments with other therapies, the first being a practical one. If we have given a Bowen treatment and then give a massage, reflexology treatment, or whatever, how can we then manage the outcomes? If the client has an exceedingly positive response, how do we duplicate the conditions? The danger then comes that we are thinking: "Gosh, this works better when I put a bit of this or that in on top."

On the other hand what about when the opposite happens? With Bowen, the client may have some strong reactions and if this happens and we have added other therapies, what is it that we need to do to handle it? Indeed can we be sure that it is a reaction to the Bowen, the other treatment or the combination given?

If the client has gone to another therapist, we have no idea what that therapist has done and are in the position that it is impossible to give reliable advice.

The main reason, however, that we strongly avoid other treatments is that it has the effect of wiping out or at best altering the effect. We need to remember that we are trying to encourage a communication between body and brain based around subtle muscle moves. The technique is not in effect just during the session time, but carries on over the period of the following week or ten days.

It's a little like listening to a radio. The equipment is capable of receiving hundreds of different signals, but you can only listen to one station at a time. If you try getting more than one, you end up with interference and distortion. It is important to explain in advance to the client the importance of not introducing other treatments, especially as the first response of a client, when reacting to Bowen, is to run off to the doctor or chiropractor.

Other Factors to Consider

No Result?

As with any treatment, there are no guarantees of success. In many cases however, the therapist can increase the odds of success by looking at a few reasons why clients might not be showing the improvement that perhaps they could. There are three areas that should be explored in the event of lack of success.

1. You

It's important when trying to establish an outcome that you look at what it is you are judging. Some therapists will view a set of treatments as having failed, simply because they are viewing the outcome from a personal perspective.

Notes are an important element of treatment and an area that many therapists fall down on. Most people cannot remember pain and so if there is insufficient information in the notes to make an effective comparison from one week to the next, then it will be easy to miss significant changes.

Other things that the therapist should look at are: have you done enough or perhaps too much; have you asked the right questions and interpreted the answers correctly (in effect how well are you listening to what is being said to you).

2. The Client

The major area of clients not responding is that of re-injury and, although this might seem to be obvious, a lot of people will re-injure without even being aware that they have. This subconscious re-injury can come in three major but not exclusive groups:

1. Conscious re-injury of the same or different area previously injured
2. Subconscious re-injury of the same or different area
3. Postural or habitual injury

Someone who has presented with a strain to the hamstring and after treatment plays a game of football where he gets kicked or falls, is going to be conscious of the fact that he has sustained either a fresh injury or has exacerbated the original problem. Remember that the one-week rule is abandoned here and the client should be re-treated as soon as possible after the re-injury has occurred.

It can be easy for someone with an imbalance or weakness to re-injure themselves and be totally unaware that they have done so. A trip or a pull or a way of performing a task can be enough to 'put out' a weak area. A good example of this is the client who presented with a shoulder strain. After two treatments the shoulder was giving him no problem at all and he was discharged. Three weeks later he called again to say that it was back to square one. Puzzled, I expressed my certainty that he must have done something to re-injure himself but he assured me that this wasn't the case. After some more discussion it transpired that he had been walking the usually very placid dog, when a cat had crossed their path and the dog had tried to go for it. Fortunately it was on the lead and although small, gave a significant enough pull on the recovering shoulder, to stop the progress that had been made.

The incident was so casual to my client that he needed quite some prompting before recalling it, even though he did note at the time that he had felt a twinge of pain in the shoulder.

The third area can also be one where some detective work is required. Even the most mundane of jobs or tasks can lead to a strain or pain, if done badly. Repetitive Strain Injury (RSI) is not something in which I hold much faith, but there is no doubt that poor working practices can lead to injury. Sitting in an awkward position, particularly when driving, is another source of many problems and I even witnessed one client who had a habit of slightly jumping her chair forward as she sat down. It wasn't a big movement, but it was enough to jar her back and slow her progress with the treatment. It's worth taking some time to play Sherlock Holmes and find out what might be stopping the full recovery.

3. Does the Client Want to Recover?

Finally when all else has failed and we have clearly not made the progress that would be indicated, we have to ask a difficult question. Does the client have an investment in their illness, disease or injury, which gives a greater return than any cure or resolution would.

By this I mean whether the client feels that there is more to be gained by not having a resolution to their particular set of problems. It might be easy to say: "They don't want to get better," but this would be little short of insulting to many people who have come to the therapist in the first place. For some people their whole life is structured around and determined by the nature of their illness and any major change, even perhaps for the better, would represent an unacceptable shift in both state of mind and practicality.

This investment might be financial, or it might be emotional whereby an individual is receiving the support and care that they would not otherwise have. It's a contentious issue and not something that can be looked at in depth here, but these situations can and do arise.

Working With Children

Bowen on children is particularly rewarding as they tend to respond very quickly and have none of the usual expectations and attitudes that come with being grown up.

The major difference between treating adults and children is that children tend to need much less in the way of moves, in order to prompt a response. Another element is the practical one, as it is unwise to try and leave a small child alone in a room for a two-minute break. A session with a child will tend to be much shorter than with an adult, the exception being the first treatment, when I will spend some time chatting to the child and the parent in order to build some kind of picture about them. After that, however, the treatments will be around ten or fifteen minutes in length and have very few moves.

With a small child I will rarely put them up on a treatment bed or couch, but will treat them on the floor, whilst they are playing. The major rule however is to never treat a child without another adult in the room, preferably a parent or guardian. For the purposes of law, a child refers to a minor or someone under the age of sixteen.

It's also worth pointing out a less known area of law, which states that a parent with a sick child who does not seek qualified medical advice is committing an offence. Not much a therapist can do here except recognise where the role of complementary medicine begins and ends.

Children tend to present less with the aches and pains that trouble adults, but will quite often have problems that are more organic in nature, such as asthma, glue ear, colic in babies, bedwetting etc. All of these problems respond well to Bowen and, with children, outcomes tend to be much clearer without the scepticism with which adults can convince themselves that nothing is changing.

Vaccinations

One of the major presentations with children is post-vaccination syndrome, where normally healthy children have had their immune system obliterated by a pointless vaccine. I have long questioned the wisdom of bombarding a developing immune system with dozens of chemicals that don't actually give lifelong immunity. There is considerable weight to the argument that the increase in asthma, cancer and the massive decline in the human immune system as well as other problems such as MS and ME are as a direct result of the vaccination programme. This has treated children as little more than laboratory guinea pigs over the last forty years. I am convinced that we are heading for a disaster which has already started and which will see simple diseases create havoc in our society as the immune system, obliterated by overuse of drugs and vaccines, gives way.

For me this is a lot more than theory, as my wife and I have had to make decisions about whether to have our two children vaccinated. After a lot of extensive reading and research, our feeling was that ultimately the vaccination programme is little more than a massive experiment that has a potentially dangerous outcome. As a result we decided to spare our children's immune systems from the onslaught that was, with little or no scientific justification, being suggested.

Working With Animals

As for working with children, The Bowen Technique is highly effective for working with animals of any size. There are established courses run by two people in the UK teaching people to use Bowen on horses. Any properly run course for horses will always insist that the practitioner learns human

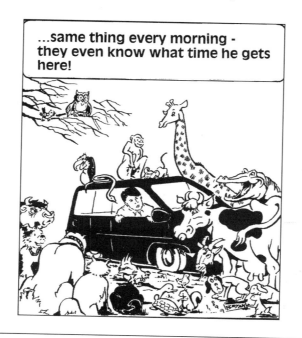

...same thing every morning - they even know what time he gets here!

Bowen first as many, if not most, horse injuries are exacerbated or caused by postural problems with the rider, which have to be addressed first.

Dogs and cats also respond very well to Bowen moves and, at one place I visit, the dog will come and sit on my feet until I give him some Bowen moves, after which he will happily get up and walk away. Animals instinctively know what is good for them and need very little work in order to restore their equilibrium.

In the UK, however, the law is tricky when it comes to working on animals and as such states that any animal (even your own) cannot be treated without the consent of a veterinary surgeon. I would think that it's unlikely that giving your dog a few Bowen moves would result in a police raid, but it's just as well to be aware. The law might be an ass, but if it were it couldn't get a Bowen treatment without the vet's say so.

Diet and Exercise

A strange element within modern medicine is the one by which doctors have virtually no training in anything but the most basic outline of the importance of nutrition on health. The result is that advice on diet in order to prevent or fight illness is rarely given. The irony is that the man who coined the phrase "you are what you eat" was Hippocrates, the same man whose name is given to the Hippocratic oath. What he actually said was, "let food be your medicine and let medicine be your food." Even better.

There are many facets to diet and exercise and with the exception of a few basic rotational exercises and some foods and activities to avoid in certain circumstances, I believe that it is best to refer clients to practitioners who can give them sound and extensive advice. Having mentioned the exceptions, I should say that we advise parents of children who are bedwetting to avoid giving the children apples, pears and anything with malic acid, as it is thought that this can affect the nerve endings of the bladder. The other area is that of dairy produce, which on the whole is not a great thing to have in the diet anyway, due to the difficulty that the human digestive system has in breaking down lactose. In particular, anyone with any form of respiratory illness or congestion should definitely avoid dairy. Incidentally, dairy also includes whey powders, butter, fats and other ingredients, which are often added to products to enrich the flavour.

Nutritional advice is one of those areas where everyone has an opinion but few have any real training, myself included. As a result, a client can be on the receiving end of dozens of pieces of advice, some of which might even be totally inappropriate for them. With this in mind, I try wherever possible to refer to a qualified nutritionist.

Light Clothing

One of the features of The Bowen Technique is that it can very easily be performed through a single layer of light clothing, without losing any of its efficacy or power. The move remains the same and the brain is prompted to respond in exactly the same way. In some cases the client who doesn't have to remove their clothes is even more relaxed and comfortable with the session than they would be in their underwear.

For a lot of people the main reason they come to Bowen is this very reason, especially elderly people or people with eating disorders. Some therapists, however, prefer to work on skin and, as a compromise, my advice is that the client should always be given the choice as to whether they remove their clothing or not.

As with anything, light clothing needs to be defined, probably in advance of the session, in order to avoid jeans, heavy jumpers, and other unsuitable clothing being worn.

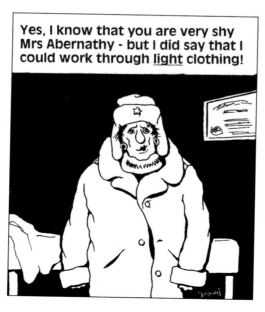

Chapter 4
Procedures of The Bowen Technique

The introduction to the technique begins with three procedures that effectively cover the whole body and pretty much encompass the initial treatment that most people would experience. Even experienced therapists will find that most of the work that they do is based around the first 3 'Pages' of work. In some Bowen circles these are referred to as basic or relaxation moves but, whilst convenient, I think this undermines the immensity of the power and effectiveness of these procedures.

We have already mentioned that The Bowen Technique works on many different levels, but it is probably best to address each procedure from a more mechanical aspect. The first set of moves works across the lower back, legs and knees. The second addresses the upper and middle back and shoulders, and the third works around the neck.

The first of these three initial procedures is often used as a prerequisite to other moves but, performed as a treatment in itself, there is little that it does not have the potential to address. The majority of clients presenting for The Bowen Technique for the first time will experience what we refer to as Pages 1, 2, 3. Quite apart from these being the first three procedures that we learn, they also represent the fact that, when we have covered these, we have thoroughly introduced the client to Bowen. 'i's dotted, 't's crossed!

I have tried to come up with some kind of snappy name such as Bowen Body Balance or BBB, but truth to tell, thousands of Bowen therapists around the world talk simply about Pages 1, 2 and 3 and know exactly what they mean. So we'll stick with 1, 2, and 3 for now.

There are few people who do not have some kind of response to Pages 1, 2, and 3 and in many cases even chronic and longstanding pain or problems have been known to be completely resolved. The most common presentation for Bowen is probably back pain and in my experience over eighty per cent of those presenting with back pain will experience significant reduction in symptoms in the first week following the application of Page 1.

Note-taking

Taking effective notes is one of the most powerful tools available to the complementary and alternative medicine therapist and also one of the areas in which even experienced therapists often fall down.

When taking notes it is important to use words that are quantifiable and therefore comparable from one week to the next. Many clients will present with diagnosed conditions, but as therapists looking at the broad picture, it is important that we don't get too focussed on one particular area. With any condition there will be variations from one person to the other. We all get sick or injured, but it is the attitude and state of mind that can often determine how quickly there will be a response.

Words such as better, worse, pain, stiffness, sore and stressed, don't really mean much by themselves. Therefore if we are talking about pain, the information we need is what kind of pain, how often, what intensity and variation, and is there any referred pain. Perhaps a scale of 1–10, with one hardly feeling the pain, and ten being absolute agony.

If there is stiffness or limitation of movement then we need to get some sort of measurement and description. Perhaps it prevents the client from performing some activity or disturbs their sleep. From this, all that is required is to get the same information from one week to the next and simply compare what is said. In this way, it is the client who is more able to judge objectively what improvement has been effected.

1. LOWER BACK AND LEGS PROCEDURE (Page 1)

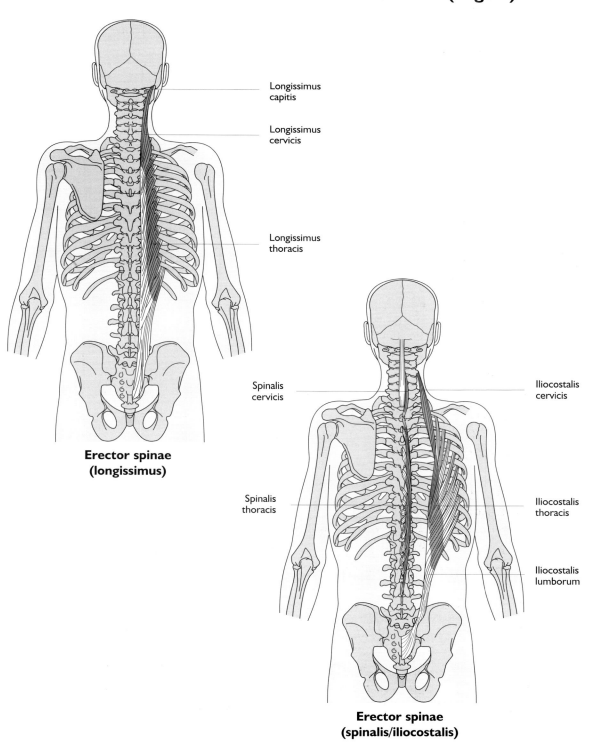

Longissimus capitis

Longissimus cervicis

Longissimus thoracis

**Erector spinae
(longissimus)**

Spinalis cervicis

Spinalis thoracis

Iliocostalis cervicis

Iliocostalis thoracis

Iliocostalis lumborum

**Erector spinae
(spinalis/iliocostalis)**

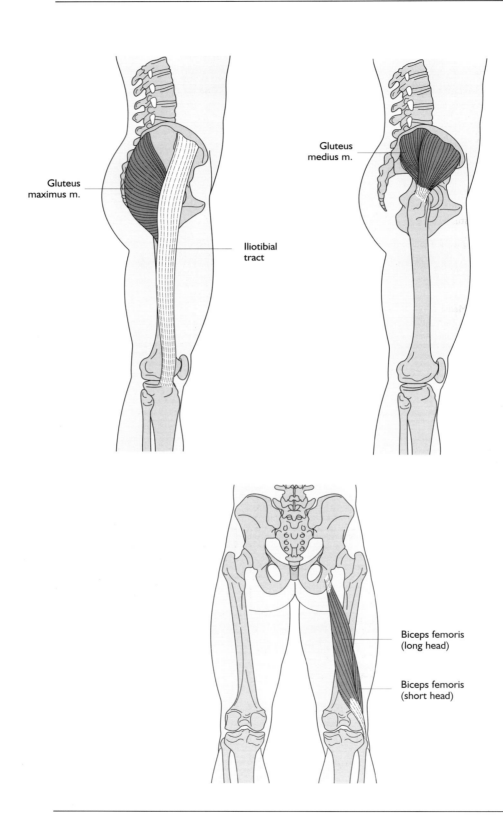

Gluteus
maximus m.

Iliotibial
tract

Gluteus
medius m.

Biceps femoris
(long head)

Biceps femoris
(short head)

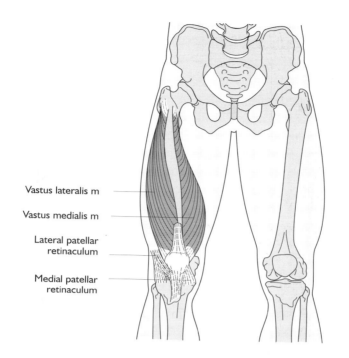

Vastus lateralis m

Vastus medialis m

Lateral patellar
retinaculum

Medial patellar
retinaculum

Muscles Worked
Erector spinae, gluteus maximus
and medius, iliotibial band (ITB),
biceps femoris, vastus lateralis.

Possible Indications for Use
Lower back pain, legs, knees, all
areas around lower back including
internal organs.

**In Conjunction with
Other Procedures**
Hamstring, knee, ankle, coccyx,
pelvic, sacrum.

Cautions or Special Notes
Can be done in a chair if client
unable to lie prone. Includes a
supine knee move to complete
the procedure.

Moves 1 and 2

Bowen moves are always performed from the left side of the client, unless otherwise specified. In many cases where we are working with specific problems, we will treat the better side first and if in doubt or if the pain or problem is central, then the left will be the side of preference. The reason for this is that the left is seen as a negative or earthing side and the right as positive. This can be seen in many approaches and also in arterial blood supply, left in right out.

The first two moves are the stoppers that we have already talked about. As well as being stoppers they also perform the function of starting to relax the whole of the body. They are both medial moves and are located slightly above the iliac crest approximately 3cms from the spinous process. Move 1 is performed with the thumbs, whilst Move 2 is done with the index fingers, with the therapist remaining standing on the left of the client.

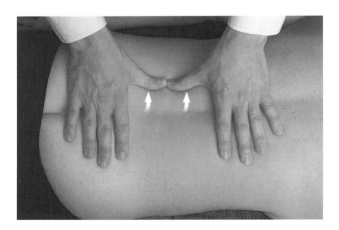

◄ *Figure 1*
The skin slack is drawn laterally.

► *Figure 2*
The thumbs roll medially.

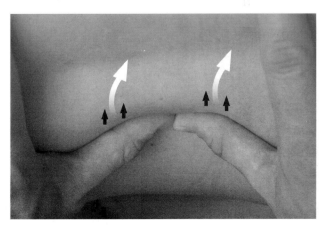

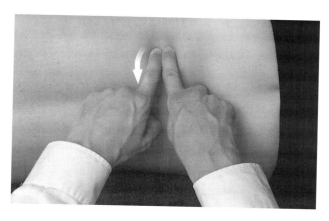

◀ *Figure 3*
The fingers move
medially on the
right side.

There is no need for the therapist to walk around the table to perform moves on the right unless this is indicated. The hands should not be rigid when using Bowen but relaxed yet controlled, allowing the hands to lift and the thumbs to roll and in turn, the fingers to draw in medially and flatten, letting the muscle move away from the direction of the move itself.

Two Minute Break

Moves 3 and 4

Moves 3 and 4 locate an overlap of gluteus medius and gluteus maximus where a small ridge or lump can be felt with palpation. These moves are an excellent point to take as a reference as they are repeated at the end of Page 1 and any changes in the tissue tension will be easy to note. Indeed especially where there is tightness or soreness in this area, it is highly likely that within a few minutes the tissue will soften and feel less tender. Move 3 is performed whilst standing on the left side but the therapist must walk around to the right side of the client for the 4th Move.

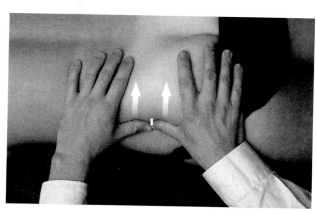

◀ *Figure 4*
Move 3, Page 1.

Moves 3 and 4 differ from Moves 1 and 2 in as much as we are working over an area with a much greater volume of tissue and will therefore find it difficult to get a roll. If we therefore imagine a cross that is drawn two finger widths above the gluteal crease and from there a straight line is drawn to the side of the body. The point we are looking for is two thirds of the way along this line towards the side of the client, on the coronal plane.

With both thumbs on this point the therapist applies eyeball type pressure and pushes slightly towards the cross above the gluteal crease, whilst slightly lifting the wrists to allow the muscle to move under the thumbs.

Two Minute Break

As mentioned earlier, it is important that the therapist informs the client that they will be leaving the room. Check that they understand this and ask if they are comfortable with this arrangement.

When coming back into the room, the therapist should avoid any unnecessary chatter or conversation, although feedback on the treatment or any experience that the client is having can be extremely valuable. Many clients will report that it felt like your hands were still on their body, or that they felt tingling, warmth, 'pins and needles' or simply just a great sense of relaxation. The therapist will make notes on anything that is said.

Moves 5–8

The next set of moves involves another feature of Bowen – that of 'holding points'. A holding point is similar to a stopper except that instead of having a lasting effect, the holding point lasts only as long as the therapist has his or her fingers in place. A holding point creates a diversion or displacement, which allows the therapist to redirect the move to another area. Whenever there is a holding point, there is always an accompanying move that corresponds to it and also always a feeling that is generated by the move and felt at the holding point. Initially these very subtle feelings are very difficult to pinpoint, but with practise become often quite marked.

In this instance the move is across the back of the knee, the popliteal fossa. It also takes in the bladder meridian, the releasing of which is what gives us our feeling. Caution should be exercised here, as a move over the adjacent biceps femoris tendon will give a similar but false reading.

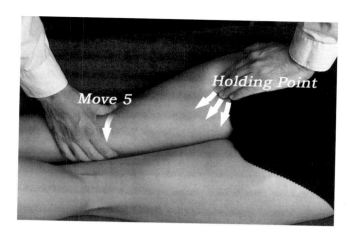

Move 5

Holding Point

◄ Figure 5
Showing
Move 5 and
holding point.

The fingers of the left hand locate the ischial tuberosity and apply gentle downward pressure onto the long head of the biceps femoris. The fingers of the right hand rest on the medial side of the leg and the thumb sits in the centre of the popliteal fossa, approximately three finger widths above the bend of the leg. The thumb takes skin slack laterally until it can feel the inside edge of the biceps femoris tendon, then applying gentle pressure, makes a medial move across the soft tissue of the popliteal fossa. The fingers of the left hand remain stationary, but the therapist should concentrate hard on trying to feel the slight blip under the fingers.

Move 6 is across the iliotibial band (ITB) slightly overlapping the vastus lateralis. This point is found approximately where the end of the client's middle finger reaches. The thumbs sit on the ITB and draw gentle pressure anteriorly. The move is a posterior move, lifting the wrists and allowing the thumbs to roll, as before. Moves 7 and 8 are performed on the right side after the therapist has walked around the treatment table.

Two Minute Break

Moves 9 and 10 finish the prone work on 'Page 1' and as already mentioned, are an ideal point at which to take stock and see what's going on. Moves 9 and 10 are simply a repeat of Moves 3 and 4, and underline and re-emphasise the area we are working in. In addition we have the opportunity to evaluate whether there has been any change. If we have focussed on the tissue tension of the client when we did the moves the first time, then we should notice that there have been some changes. Perhaps the muscle is softer, less tender, more relaxed, warmer, etc. It takes time for the therapist to learn to notice changes, but by focussing on each move as it is performed it will quickly become apparent that things are happening.

Turn Client Over

On turning the client, two small but very powerful moves are made on the lateral insertion of the vastus lateralis tendon, next to the patella. On the left side first, locate the medial edge of the patella and feel for a small ridge adjacent to it. The thumbs should move together and having taken the skin slack, roll the vastus lateralis tendon very slowly medially. This move should take at least six seconds and effectively relaxes the knee and also brings together the whole of the initial procedures that have been performed. Right side follows.

2. UPPER AND MIDDLE BACK AND SHOULDERS PROCEDURE (Page 2)

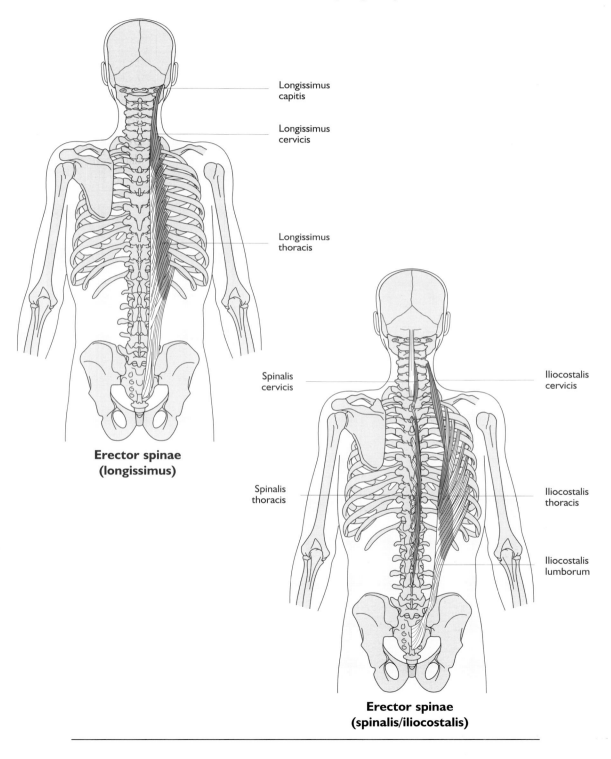

**Erector spinae
(longissimus)**

Longissimus capitis

Longissimus cervicis

Longissimus thoracis

Spinalis cervicis

Spinalis thoracis

Iliocostalis cervicis

Iliocostalis thoracis

Iliocostalis lumborum

**Erector spinae
(spinalis/iliocostalis)**

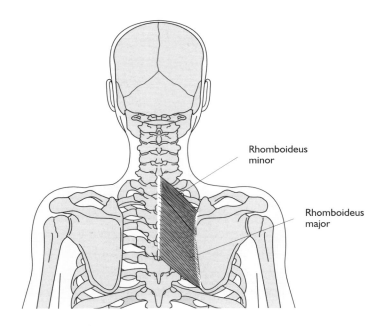

Rhomboideus
minor

Rhomboideus
major

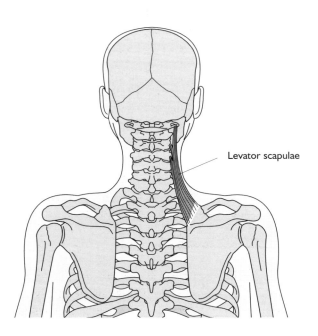

Levator scapulae

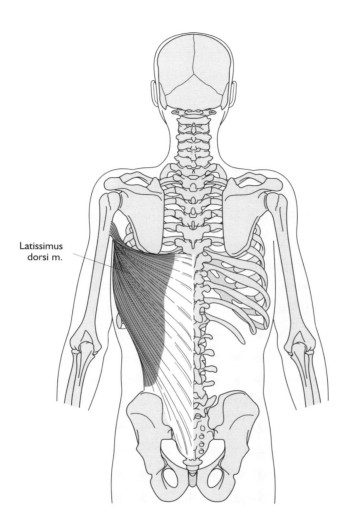

Latissimus dorsi m.

Muscles Worked
Erector spinae, rhomboid major and minor, levator scapulae, latissimus dorsi.

Possible Indications for Use
Relaxation for back and neck, whiplash, frozen shoulder, RSI, tenosinovitis, asthma, scoliosis.

In Conjunction with Other Procedures
TMJ, asthma, pelvic, shoulder, elbow, wrist, Page 3, (neck).

Cautions or Special Notes
Relaxation for back and neck, whiplash, frozen shoulder, RSI, tenosynovitis, asthma, scoliosis.

When people used to having massage first see Bowen, they often feel that it will not be as effective as lying down for a whole hour and being worked over. True there is nothing quite as nurturing as being wrapped in warm towels and pampered with nice smelling oils. For effectiveness however, there is little that comes close to Bowen, and this procedure demonstrates this highly effectively.

The human head weighs something in the region of 5kgs and needs a tremendous set of muscles to keep it held in place. Many of these muscles extend right down the thoracic spine and although we can generally localise a stiff neck, in many cases the problem will stem a long way down the spine into the mid thoracic spine.

Page 2 is ideal for any neck and shoulder problems and whereas Page 1 can be done alone, Page 2 is always done together with the 3rd Page of work. As with the lower back work, this procedure, together with the neck, often forms the prerequisite for other procedures to follow, although they are certainly effective enough to stand alone.

Moves 1–4

The first four moves are virtually identical to the lower stoppers, simply performed higher. The location for these is level with the inferior angle of the scapulae. Draw an imaginary line across the upper back level with the bottom edges of the scapulae. Moves 1 and 2 are made just below this line, with 3 and 4 slightly above. Again the skin is drawn in the opposite direction to the move and the pressure is applied only in order to make the rolling action over the muscle. Left side first.

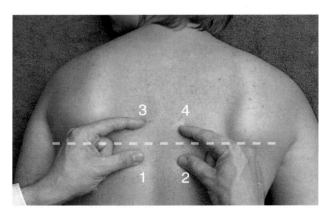

◄ *Figure 6*
Showing position
of upper stoppers.

Two Minute Break

Moves 5–8

Standing on the left side, place the fingers of the left hand on the trapezius, allowing the left thumb to sit a third of the way down the margin of the client's left scapula. The right index finger is next to it.

The thumb and fingers then apply gentle pressure and perform a semi-circular move around the rhomboideus major, coming to rest back on the scapula adjacent to the superior medial angle of the scapula. The thumb pressure is now lifted to allow the gathered skin to be released.

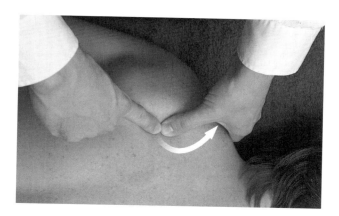

◄ *Figure 7*
Showing Move
around scapula to
find 'ladybird'.

The thumb and finger now follow the shape of the scapula around the superior medial angle of the scapula, dropping down and rolling over the levator scapulae. At this point a crunching sensation can often be felt and this is referred to as 'the ladybird'. Right side follows, for which the moves can be done from either side.

Moves 9–12

These are energetic and stimulatory moves that are performed in pairs in between the lower and upper stoppers. Move 9 is medial and is virtually identical to the lower stoppers, but simply slightly superior. Number 10's are lateral moves and differ from previous moves in as much as the left-sided move is done with the fingers and the right with the thumbs. This is

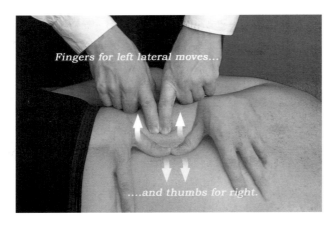

◄ *Figure 8*
For Moves 9-12.

because of the nature of the move that makes an effective and controlled lateral move virtually impossible with the thumbs.

Moves 3a and 4a

These are very effective and incredibly simple moves that add on to the upper back work, but are also a treatment in their own right. Moves 3a and 4a work on the latissimus dorsi, which broadens out from the side of the body and goes down all the way to the sacrum. At the top, its attachment to the humerus means that these moves can be very useful for a wide range of problems, including indications as diverse as frozen shoulder and asthma, the latissimus dorsi being an accessory muscle of respiration.

When making the move, the latissimus dorsi can be located level with the edge of the scapulae on the side or coronal plane of the body. There is generally a fair amount of adipose tissue in this area and this needs to be

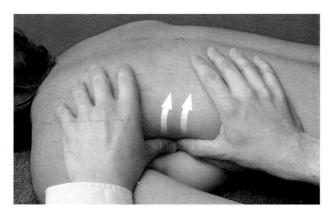

◄ *Figure 9*
Showing latissimus dorsi 3a and 4a.

moved anteriorly in order to locate the muscle, which can be compared to a sausage. Using the thumbs, the therapist takes the tissue and skin anteriorly to catch the latissimus dorsi. The move is a lifting type roll posteriorly and towards the edge of the scapula. As with the other upper back moves, the right side can be done with the therapist standing on either side. These moves are also optional and are often performed in conjunction with the moves already performed on the upper back in order to add further assistance. The neck procedures on Page 3 always follow the upper back Page 2 moves.

3. NECK MOVES PROCEDURE (Page 3)

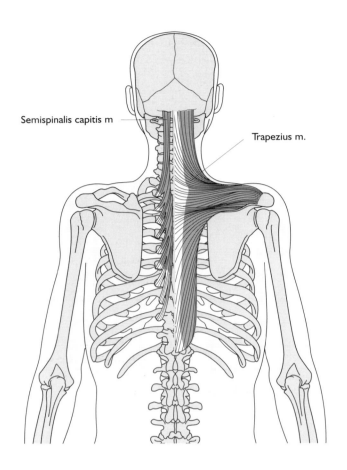

Semispinalis capitis m

Trapezius m.

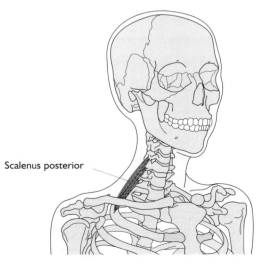

Scalenus posterior

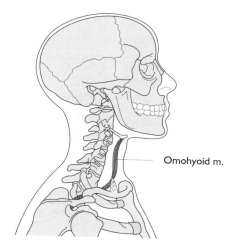

Omohyoid m.

Muscles Worked Trapezius, semispinalis capitis, scalenus posterior, border of omohyoid.	**Possible Indications for Use** Whiplash injuries, rye neck, shoulder and elbow problems, jaw and head.
In Conjunction with Other Procedures Page 2, shoulders, TMJ, elbow.	**Cautions or Special Notes** Should be preceded by Page 2. Ensure client comfort.

The client should be lying supine (face-up) and should be comfortable. If necessary a pillow or cushion can be placed under the client's head, although this should be avoided unless absolutely essential. If the client's head tilts backwards, then a small folded towel under the back of the head will bring it level and ease the location of Moves 3 and 4.

Moves 1–4

Sitting or standing at the head of the client, the therapist places the left thumb into a hollow that can be found at the base of the neck, anterior to the trapezius. The thumb is pulled around the scalenus muscles by the therapist gripping the fingers and performing a rolling action with the thumb. Once again the move is gentle and should not result in any flicking of the muscle. Right side follows.

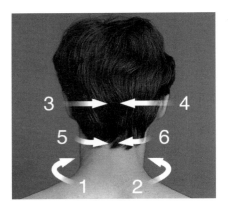

◀ *Figure 10*
Showing neck Moves.

Moves 3 and 4 are very small medial moves which affect the semispinalis capitis. The therapist locates the small knobbly protrusion at the back of the head, the occipital protuberance. By moving slightly down and medially from this point, a small wire shaped muscle can be found. This point is often quite tender and can even be swollen and hot and this indicates a degree of toxicity in the system, especially where the client drinks a lot of coffee or takes an excess of dairy products. The move is with the middle finger and is a medial move, left first followed by right. A two-minute break follows, although the power of Moves 3 and 4 suggests that a break of at least four or five minutes would be more appropriate.

Moves 5 and 6

These moves are in principle identical to the moves performed on the spine with the client prone. The client is still supine and the therapist performs the moves with the middle finger, taking skin slack laterally, applying gentle pressure and performing a medial rolling move over the trapezius, on the centre of the back of the neck, halfway between Moves 1 and 4.

Most busy Bowen therapists will tell you that these three procedures form the majority of the work that they do and the efficacy and power of these Pages should not be underestimated. At first the common reaction from therapists seeing the work for the first time is: "Is that all there is to it?" Each move is performed once only, although with experience the therapist will discover where additional moves can be performed. The client too is often surprised at how minimal the treatment is, especially if they have been used to chiropractic or other treatments where more is done and greater pressure used. The simplicity of Bowen is its key, both in its ease of application and its efficacy.

The examples of Bowen are given in this book in order to demonstrate the range of moves that a basic Bowen course will teach, but are by no means comprehensive. As I have already mentioned, The Bowen Technique is not simply a series of documented techniques, but a philosophy of body repair, with clearly defined parameters and principles. Within these principles there are literally millions of different combinations of moves and sequences of which the following are simply examples.

ANKLE PROCEDURE

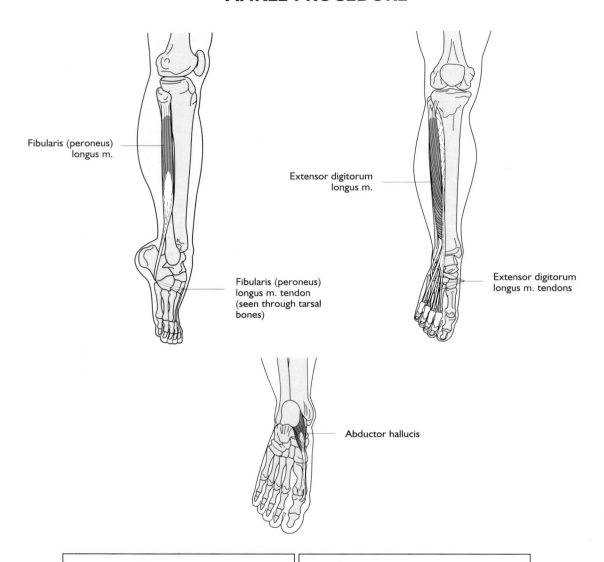

Fibularis (peroneus) longus m.

Extensor digitorum longus m.

Fibularis (peroneus) longus m. tendon (seen through tarsal bones)

Extensor digitorum longus m. tendons

Abductor hallucis

Muscles Worked
Abductor hallucis, peroneus longus, extensor digitorum longus, deltoid ligament.

Possible Indications for Use
Sprained ankles, (even acute) swellings in the feet, foot and toe problems, knee pain.

In Conjunction with Other Procedures
Page 1 hamstring, knee, pelvic.

Cautions or Special Notes
Any acute injury should be X-rayed and examined by a doctor.

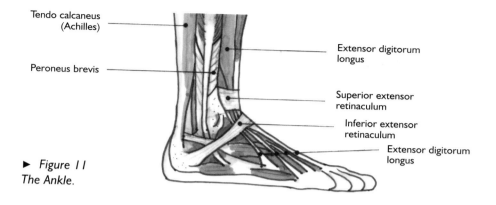

Tendo calcaneus
(Achilles)

Peroneus brevis

Extensor digitorum
longus

Superior extensor
retinaculum

Inferior extensor
retinaculum

Extensor digitorum
longus

▶ Figure 11
The Ankle.

The ankle procedure has on occasion been seen to be little short of miraculous in addressing the acute pain of a twisted or sprained ankle and demonstrates why Bowen in acute situations is such an effective tool. As with any trauma to a joint or where sharp pain is present, the client should be referred to a hospital for X-ray. If there are no fractures or breaks, then this work can be done, but naturally with care.

The work can be done with the client sitting or lying. The therapist positions himself with the inside or medial aspect of the ankle facing him, the calf resting on the therapists' leg, with the heel free. The moves indicated here are for the left foot.

Moves 1–3

The right hand pushes the foot into gentle dorsiflexion, while the left hand makes the moves.

The 1st Move is medial, made with the index finger across the extensor digitorum longus, with the skin slack being first taken in the opposite direction.

Move 2 has two sections to it and is in the form of a T or a cross, moving initially over the lateral malleolus and ending inferior to the talofibular ligament. The index finger starts on the top of the lateral malleolus and makes an inferior move, with the side of the finger finishing under the heel bone and resting lightly on the skin. The finger then draws the skin slack anteriorly and applies gentle pressure, before moving posteriorly over the peroneus longus towards the Achilles tendon.

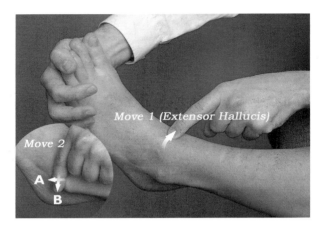
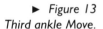

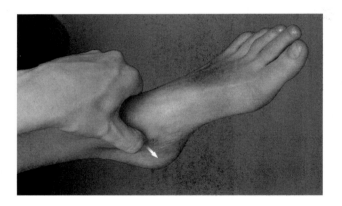

◀ *Figure 12*
Ankle Moves
1 and 2.

The 3rd Move is with the thumb and is a diagonal move over the fibres of the deltoid ligament, towards the heel.

▶ *Figure 13*
Third ankle Move.

With the finger and thumb resting forward of points two and three, the right hand holding around the metatarsal pad now rotates the foot erratically in different directions. This is done in order to relax the foot and confuse the brain from setting up a pattern. When the foot is sufficiently relaxed the therapist pushes the metatarsal pad sharply into flexion and at the same time pushes inwards and downwards with the left thumb and finger, towards the heel.

As with any acute or painful area, the pressure of the moves should be adjusted to ensure that no pain is experienced with the treatment. Any continued pain or swelling should be dealt with using apple cider vinegar or washing soda as required (see pages 141–142). Strapping may also be required in order to maintain support and control over the ankle area.

ASTHMA/RESPIRATORY PROCEDURE

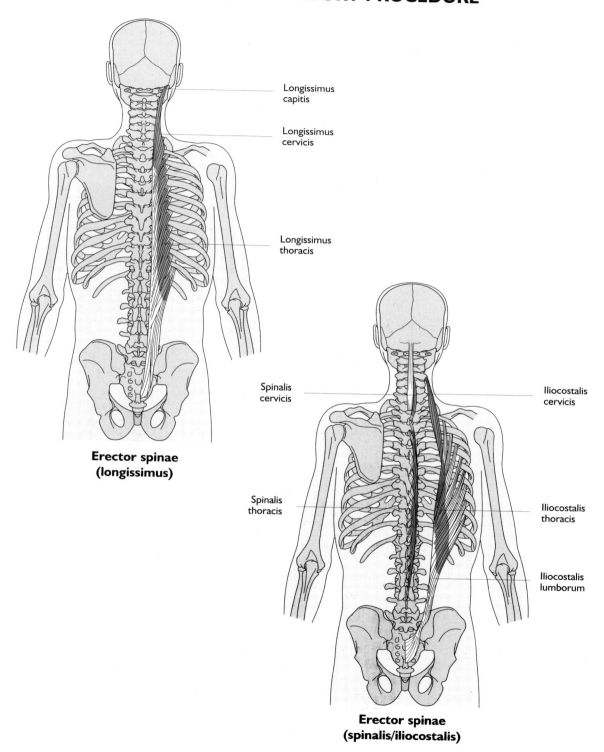

Longissimus
capitis

Longissimus
cervicis

Longissimus
thoracis

**Erector spinae
(longissimus)**

Spinalis
cervicis

Spinalis
thoracis

Iliocostalis
cervicis

Iliocostalis
thoracis

Iliocostalis
lumborum

**Erector spinae
(spinalis/iliocostalis)**

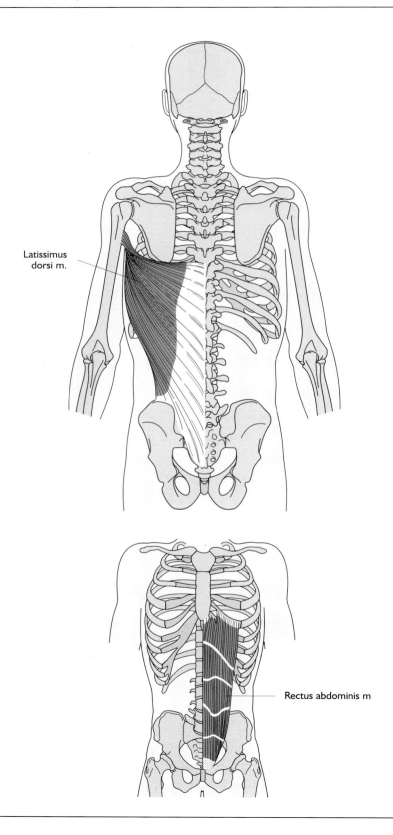

Latissimus
dorsi m.

Rectus abdominis m

Muscles Worked	Possible Indications for Use
Latissimus dorsi, erector spinae, rectus abdominis.	Asthma, respiratory illness, chest pain, digestion problems.
In Conjunction with Other Procedures Pages 1, 2 and 3, TMJ coccyx, breast	**Cautions or Special Notes** Not a substitute for medical treatment. Anyone having an asthma attack should not be lain down.

The condition referred to as asthma has, over the last few years, grown to epidemic proportions, with people being diagnosed as asthmatic at the merest suggestion of a tight chest. These clients are then given bronchial dilators and often steroids by their GP and spend the next few years inhaling these, wondering why they feel terrible. Obviously in many cases there are people who owe their lives to the availability of these drugs, but there are undoubtedly many more, possibly the majority, who don't need them and shouldn't be on them.

There are many causes cited for asthma. Air pollution, stress, house dust mite faeces, central heating, double glazing, food additives, pesticides, vaccination. These are all possible factors that have been identified over the years, but as yet no-one has pointed the finger and no-one has come up with a cure. Little surprise given the amount of money that's involved in drug therapy but there are things that a client can do to help and even eradicate the symptoms of asthma.

The obvious include avoiding those things that exacerbate any symptoms, but a change in diet can often be very helpful. Dairy products – milk, cheese, yoghurt etc. – create a lot of mucus in the system, which combined with the use of bronchial dilators can cause big problems and eliminating dairy from the diet can be very beneficial. Anyone worried about calcium in dairy need not worry, as there is lots of available calcium in many other foods.

The asthma/respiratory procedure introduces the concept of locking areas of the body by lifting the leg. There are three procedures in this book which use this and these are respiratory, coccyx and kidney. The idea of this is to open up an area of the body that is then isolated. In effect it presents the body for the work to be done and is a powerful way of directing moves to certain areas. The principle can be applied in many ways, but these three are the most obvious for the moment. Whenever there is a lock required, there are three elements present on the same side.

1. The face of the client, turned to the side where the therapist is standing.
2. The leg lifted up from the medial aspect of the ankle to an angle of 90 degrees and allowed to drop out.
3. The therapist.

The moves for asthma aren't exclusively for asthmatics, but are used for anyone with any kind of respiratory illness. Also indigestion, liver and gall bladder can be affected by these moves.

There are two parts to the procedure, some with the client prone and some with the client supine.

Prerequisite Moves

Upper back and shoulders Page 2, Moves 1–8 also Moves 3a and 4a, latissimus dorsi, which is an accessory muscle of respiration.

Asthma/Respiratory Procedure Moves

Before turning the client, have them turn their face to the left. The left leg is lifted at right angles to the body with the therapists' right hand, ensuring the knees are together.

This is the same approach as used when working the kidney. The therapist's hand should be on the inside of the ankle applying gentle downward pressure on the ankle, to lock the mid-thoracic spine.

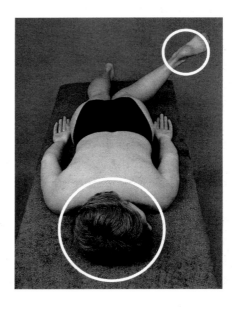

▶ *Figure 14. Client position for asthma Moves.*

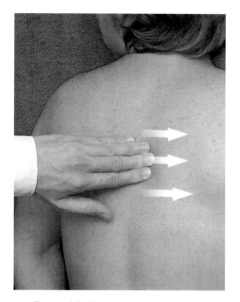

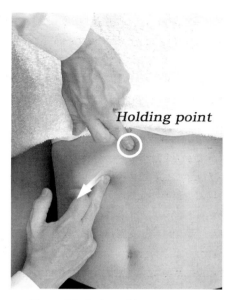

▲ Figure 15. Asthma Moves on back.

▲ Figure 16. Asthma Moves on costal margin.

NOTE: This locking movement may be seen or felt in the thoracic area at around T6/T7, but is often undetectable.

With the leg lifted and locked and with the client's head facing the therapist, a lateral move is made across the erector spinae on the opposite side, with the fingers or heel of the left hand.

This is then repeated on the right side, ensuring that the head, raised leg and therapist are on the same side. The move is made where the movement of the thoracic spine was located. If no movement was detected, the move is made on an imaginary line running between the inferior angles of both scapulae.

Turn Client

NOTE: The therapist is now halfway through the procedure, and must therefore finish the asthma procedure before any other moves are performed elsewhere.

Standing on the right hand side of the client, the therapist locates the xiphoid process at the end of the sternum, and with the middle finger of the left hand holds gently just inferior to the xiphoid process. The right thumb takes skin slack along the left costal margin superiorly towards the xiphoid.

Then on the exhalation tucks the thumb under the rib and moves laterally and slightly inferiorly over the rectus abdominis insertion, along the border of the costal margin.

Maintaining the gentle holding point at the base of the xiphoid, the middle finger of the right hand is used to make the move on the right rectus abdominis. Release the holding point.

Using the middle finger of the right hand and starting just below the holding point, the skin slack is taken up and moved inferiorly over the rectus abdominis towards the navel.

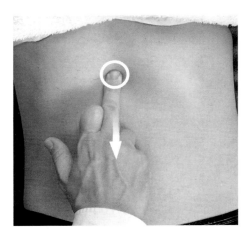

◄ *Figure 17*
Final asthma
Move.

The client can often experience slight reactions after this procedure, such as shivering or a feeling of nausea. If this occurs then they should be lain down again and kept warm, until the feeling passes. If the client does vomit then this again is no cause for alarm.

Page 3 Neck Moves 1–6, observing the two-minute breaks as directed completes this procedure.

An emergency procedure for someone having an asthma attack is to use the final move, inferior to the xiphoid process, but with the client standing. The move is made quite firmly with the thumb, and can be repeated as required.

Other variations on this procedure address chest pains and spinal deformities. There are also modified moves on the same theme that address babies with colic and asthma.

BREAST PROCEDURE

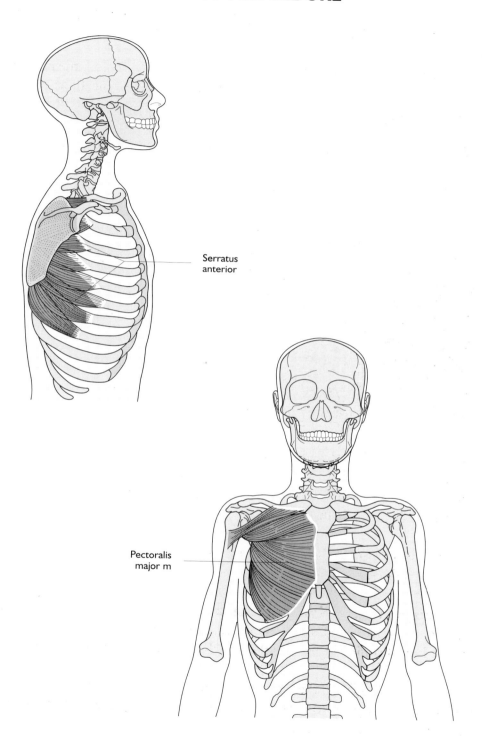

Serratus anterior

Pectoralis major m

Muscles Worked Pectoralis major, serratus anterior.	**Possible Indications for Use** Breast pain or tenderness, breast lumps, inflammation, mastitis.
In Conjunction with Other Procedures Neck move, TMJ, asthma, pelvic, shoulder, elbow, wrist, kidney, Page 3 neck.	**Cautions or Special Notes** This procedure can be self administered. **It does not require the removal of bras or light clothing.**

Every year in the UK, something like 15,000 women die of breast cancer, a rate which is one of the highest in Europe. There have been few advances in the field of cancer treatment in nearly thirty years and the death rates only rise. One of the questions that I ask women around the country is how many of them perform a thorough self-examination of their breasts every thirty days. It averages at less than ten per cent and yet early detection of any irregular lumps or bumps can be the difference between life and premature death.

For a lot of women there is a fear of finding a lump, yet in most cases lumps will be benign swellings or fatty lumps. The main issue in this area is one of lymphatics and a lot of problems could be avoided by keeping a good movement of lymph in the area around the breast. This procedure does exactly that and as a result has to be considered to be a preventative measure for congestion in the breast tissue, which can lead on to other problems.

The avoidance of underwired and tight bras, is another recommendation within the field of self-help. This move is generally taught to women to perform weekly on themselves, but it can also be given to men, who also suffer from both breast cancer and mastitis.

NOTE: The moves themselves are not invasive and do not require the therapist to touch breast tissue. Light clothing does not need to be removed and bras do not need to be adjusted, undone or removed. This should be discussed thoroughly with the client so that they understand fully what is involved.

CAUTION: Do not use this procedure on women with breast implants. This is one of the few contra-indications within Bowen and is given more as a caution than for any other reason. With the recent cases of leakage in implanted breasts, not due to Bowen, any therapist might be placed in a difficult situation legally should leakage occur after treatment.

Recommended Prerequisite Moves

Pages 1, 2 and 3.

Treat Better Side First

Breast Procedure Moves

With the client supine, the therapist stands on the opposite side to the breast being treated. A pen or pencil is placed under the client's arm, in line with the nipple or middle of the breast. (The pen is placed in line with the nipple to give a guide to the amount of breast tissue to be moved).

Treatment for Left Breast

The client is asked to place the palm of their right hand on the upper part of the breast. The therapist places their right hand on top of the client's hand. The index fingers of the therapist's right and left hands should be touching. The breast tissue is moved gently inferiorly until the index fingers are just above the line of the pen.

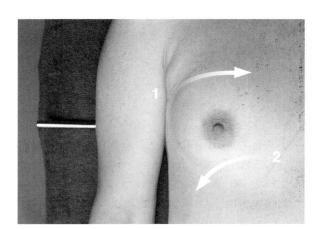

◄ *Figure 18. Positioning and directions of breast Moves.*

Skin slack is taken laterally, allowing the index finger of the left hand to curve around the pectoralis major. Gentle pressure is then applied and the move is made medially over the pectoral. Ask the client to place the palm of their right hand under the breast tissue.

The palm of the therapist's left hand now sits on top of the client's hand and gently moves the breast tissue superiorly (towards client's head) until the index fingers are just below the line of the pen OR as far as is comfortable for the client.

Taking skin slack medially, the therapist moves laterally over the projection of serratus anterior. All that can be felt on this move is skin and possibly some rib. Once again, the index fingers will be adjacent to each other.

NOTE: During this procedure, both hands move, avoiding the possibility of any friction around breast tissue.

Guidance for Patient

Instruction may be given to the client to encourage self-administration of the breast procedure. Body brushing is an ideal adjunct to the breast procedure and greatly aids the movement of lymph through the system.

COCCYX PROCEDURE

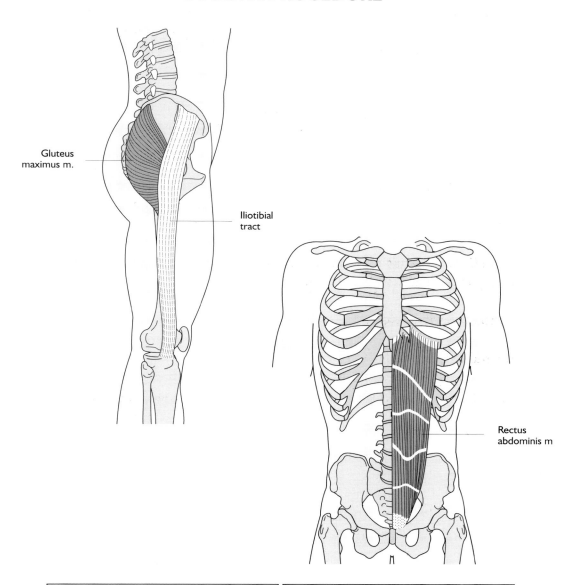

Gluteus maximus m.

Iliotibial tract

Rectus abdominis m

Muscles Worked Rectus abdominis, gluteus maximus.	**Possible Indications for Use** *see* pie chart, page 96.
In Conjunction with Other Procedures Lower back Page 1, pelvic.	**Cautions or Special Notes** Must not be performed in pregnancy.

The coccyx procedure is one of the 'big guns' of The Bowen Technique. As a procedure it affects many of the body systems and creates a strong energetic balance for the whole body. There are three major parts that we can look at when taking an overview of the coccyx procedure. Although we will look at these as particular areas, it is important to remind ourselves that the technique is a treatment for the whole body.

Reproductive

The coccyx procedure addresses both male and female reproductive systems from an energetic perspective, and allows the normal functioning of this complex system. As there are more parts to the female reproductive system, it follows that there are more potential problems. Infertility is an area that is fraught with variants and it is often wrongly thought that this is more a female problem than male. As it happens it is one of those conditions that is equally spread between male and female, and the consistent fall in male sperm counts due to synthetic materials, central heating and other factors over the last twenty years has not helped. Certain mineral deficiencies can have an effect as well and if in doubt, a consultation with a clinical nutritionist would help.

Prostate is another area where the coccyx might be useful in the male reproductive system although once again diet can have a good effect in helping to control problems in this area.

For the female reproductive system, the list of potential problems is very extensive and the coccyx procedure can be used to good effect in any of the areas of female reproductive health. It has even been reported that ovarian cysts have reduced or in some cases disappeared after Bowen treatment.

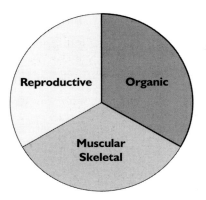

Muscular Skeletal

The coccyx is four fused bones located at the base of the spine and is often neglected in modern medicine. In many other traditions and schools of therapeutic thought, the coccyx is an important site of energetic response. In Chinese medicine the coccyx area is around the base of the Governing Vessel. In chakra work, the opening of the root or base chakra is the basis for balancing all the chakras, or energy centres, through the body. In Hindu Vedic medicine the life energy or Kundalini arises from the base of the spine and travels upwards through the chakras, aiding spiritual growth.

In terms of the purely physical, a fall or jar to the coccyx can be very painful and can lead to a lot of back problems for quite a long time. In childbirth the coccyx has to move to allow the complete opening of the birth canal. In addition the base of the spine plays an important role in the act of physical balancing, with nerve endings giving information to the inner ear.

In some cases deformed or damaged cocci are surgically removed, but a simply performed coccyx procedure can bring significant changes and avoid the need for this type of operation.

Organic

The coccyx procedure addresses the peristaltic action of the colon and is therefore very indicated in a wide range of intestinal problems. Included in this is the problem of allergic reactions arising from colonic or digestive weakness or illness. Problems such as diverticulitis, Crohn's disease, Irritable Bowel Syndrome or even simply trapped wind or stomach cramping can all be helped with the coccyx procedure.

Skin conditions are often a result of colon and bowel problems and are therefore included in this section. Migraines and even bad hay fever can be caused or exacerbated by histamine reactions in the gut. As well as performing the coccyx procedure, it is also important to address the diet and in particular the intake of dairy, refined sugar and wheat and a referral to a trained nutritionist is recommended.

The procedure itself is very slight and unlike most other Bowen procedures, is only performed on one side. Because of this the therapist needs to assess to see which side is indicated. This can be done in several ways, by feel, observation and discussion as to whether one side or the other might have any kind of tenderness.

The observation can look at several areas. Which way the gluteal crease is pointing, whether the lower back is raised or swollen on one side, the movement of the gluteal tissue on palpation, heat on one side or the other, etc.

The coccyx could be considered to be in an invasive area and for this reason, this procedure should be discussed and explained clearly before proceeding. Part of this discussion should also include the warning that the coccyx is contra-indicated in pregnancy and if a woman is or even feels that she might be pregnant, then the therapist must not proceed with the coccyx procedure.

The coccyx is the last procedure done on the back. If any other moves are needed, do these first and then come back to the coccyx.

Observation and Assessment

The stoppers should be done before assessing. The therapist feels down the coccyx to approximately halfway down the coccyx bone and touches initially VERY gently on one side of the coccyx then the other, asking the client to indicate whether one side is more tender.

If neither side is tender, then the coccyx may be touched again using slightly more pressure. If still no indication, then treat the side that has been chosen by the therapist through feeling for any deviation or observing swelling on the side of the buttocks would be treated.

If neither side is indicated by tenderness or observation, then the left side should be treated.

CAUTION: Clients with hip replacements should not have their hips pushed through 90 degrees.

Prerequisite Moves

Minimum: Page 1, Moves 1 and 2.

Coccyx Procedure Moves

Treatment for left side more tender. The therapist stands on the left of the client.

Move 1. The therapist locates the left side of the coccyx with the index finger of the left hand and feels for the lateral edge of the sacrum on the opposite side with the middle finger of the same hand.

The left leg is then lifted with the right hand and flexed to 90 degrees allowing it to drop out to the side. Gentle pressure is applied to the medial aspect of the client's ankle to lock the leg. This is identical to the locking for the asthma and kidney procedures (see figure 14).

On the exhalation of the client the skin is moved directly across the coccyx bone towards the holding point on the opposite side.

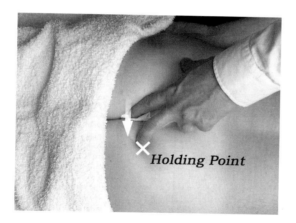

Holding Point

◄ *Figure 19*

The client should then be turned. A two-minute break here is advisable although not compulsory.

Move 2. The therapist must now go around the table and position himself on the left hand side of the client. The left leg is carried out laterally a few centimetres, so that the foot is in a line with the right shoulder.

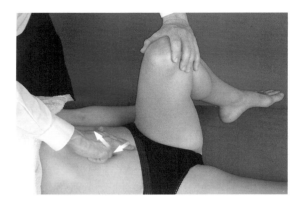

◄ *Figure 20*

Finding a point halfway between the mid-inguinal ligament and the navel, the leg is lifted and the index and middle fingers of your right hand placed on this point. Whilst carrying the knee towards the opposite shoulder, the skin slack is taken in a line down towards the inguinal ligament. Very gentle pressure is applied and a move is made towards the navel, over the rectus abdominis. When the limit of the skin has been reached, a lateral move is made as if to complete the drawing of a seven.

The knee continues to be taken and slightly pushed towards the opposite shoulder but only within the comfort of the client.

The leg and knee is straightened and lowered gently to the table, whilst being supported on the way down.

NOTE: When the coccyx procedure has been completed, any other moves required can be done whilst the client is supine.

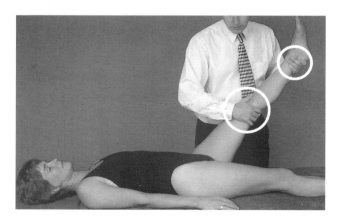

◄ *Figure 21*

ELBOW PROCEDURE

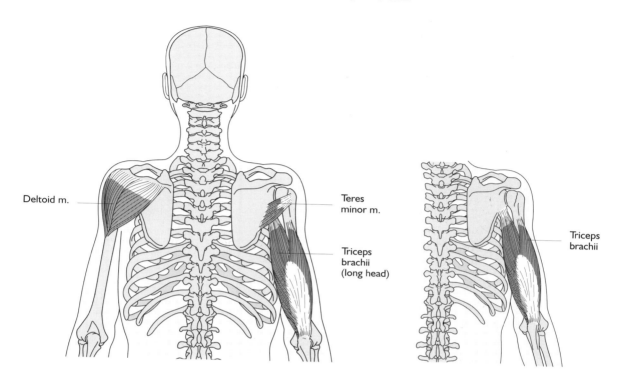

Deltoid m.

Teres
minor m.

Triceps
brachii
(long head)

Triceps
brachii

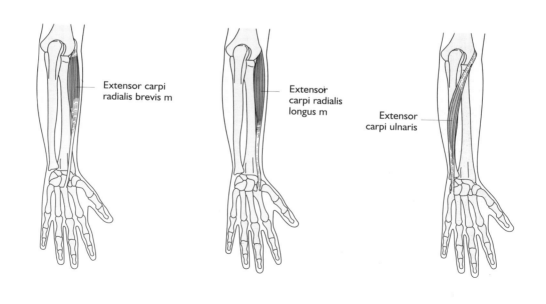

Extensor carpi
radialis brevis m

Extensor
carpi radialis
longus m

Extensor
carpi ulnaris

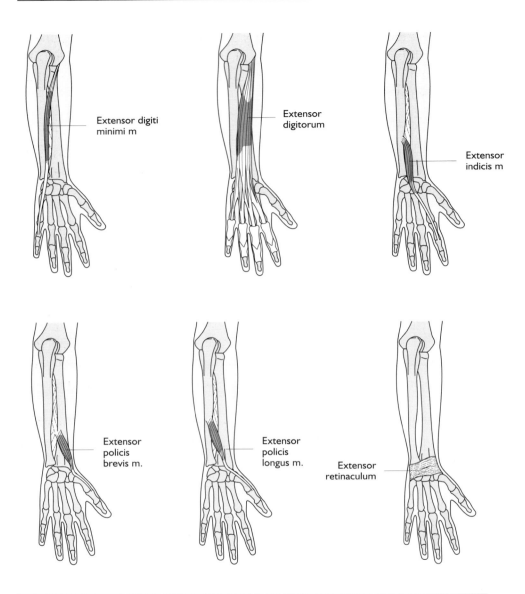

Extensor digiti minimi m

Extensor digitorum

Extensor indicis m

Extensor policis brevis m.

Extensor policis longus m.

Extensor retinaculum

Muscles Worked Deltoid, triceps, extensors of the arm, retinaculum extensors.	**Possible Indications for Use** Tennis or golfer's elbow, RSI, Carpal Tunnel Syndrome, other conditions of the hand or arm.
In Conjunction with Other Procedures Shoulder, TMJ, Pages 2 and 3 (upper back and neck).	**Cautions or Special Notes** The extension must only be performed under supervision.

The elbow procedure has a consistently good track record in treating one of the most difficult and stubborn areas. Cortisone injections are often used with shoulder and elbow complaints and although very successful in some cases, they have a poor average.

With Bowen, even a chronic elbow can be affected very quickly and there are many stories of people in sporting or working environments, whose first exposure to The Bowen Technique has been when they complained of elbow pain and were treated there and then by a keen exponent.

A friend of mine who is a keen low handicap golfer had been complaining of pain in both his elbows for some time, but kept putting off coming to see me. One day when I was coming off the golf course he was going towards the first tee and on seeing me, again complained of his elbow pain. There and then I grabbed one arm and gave it a very quick elbow treatment, with only the time to do one, as his partner was waiting for him. As he stood on the tee and hit his ball, the expected pain in one elbow did not appear and the ball flew sharply right and ended in a large pond. He had no further pain in one elbow and the other was sorted when he eventually came for a full treatment.

The elbow procedure is one of the more complex of Bowen procedures and is therefore broken down into three parts, each with three moves, to make it easier to understand.

Part 1

This procedure is best done with the client sitting on the treatment couch or in a chair. The work can also be performed with the client lying supine.

Treatment for client sitting, with right elbow being treated. The therapist stands facing the client.

Approximately three fingers inferiorly from the shoulder capsule, the therapist locates the mid-point of the deltoid with the middle or index finger of the left hand. The skin slack is taken posteriorly, pressure applied and a Bowen move made over the mid-deltoid anteriorly.

The underside of the client's forearm is then rested onto the therapists' extended fingers that are held as if playing guns. The thumb rests onto the upperside of the forearm, with the thumbnail facing the ceiling. The therapist drops the upper wrist and in so doing draws the skin. Gentle pressure is applied to the extensor with the thumb, the wrist then lifts and rolls over the extensor digitorum communis. A slight flick or movement of the client's middle finger indicates that the move has been successful.

From this position, the middle finger of the left hand moves around and locates the medial epicondyle. From the top of the epicondyle, the medial border of the triceps tendon can be located 2 centimetres superior to the epicondyle. The middle finger pushes the skin towards the client, before applying gentle pressure and rolling over the tendon away from the client.

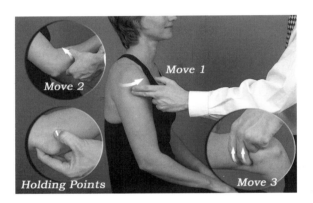

◀ *Figure 22. Elbow procedure (right side).*

Part 2

(a), (b) and (c) 'The Tripod' – are holding points. These are designed to slightly anaesthetise the elbow area, in preparation for the adjustment that will ensue. Standing directly in front of the client, the therapist supports the arm with the right hand. The index and middle fingers are drawn down the triceps in a line towards the therapist. Just before these fingers leave the client, the medial epicondyle can be located. The middle finger sits anterior to the medial epicondyle and the index finger finds soft tissue in a groove for the ulnar nerve on the outside edge of the epicondyle.

The thumb feels for a groove between the humerus and the head of the radius at the head of the radiohumeral joint. Moving the client's arm to and fro will help in the location of this. These three digits now apply increasing pressure for ten seconds or until the client reports tingling, cold, numbness or any other sensations in the forearm or fingers.

Part 3

Supporting the client's wrist with the right hand, the therapist makes a move towards the radial (thumb) side of the wrist across the extensors at the base of the wrist, using the left thumb. (This is dependent upon which side is being treated).

Holding the wrist between the thumbs and index fingers of both hands with the rest of the fingers supporting the palm of the client's hand, the wrist is extended by pushing the thumbs and pulling with the fingers. The wrist is rotated in a figure of eight motion being careful not to allow the wrist to drop down. Ensuring that the arm is relaxed, a gentle flick is performed, with a simultaneous slight pull of the arm.

The client must now extend the wrist and arm away, 'The Snake'. This is done slowly at first and with assistance, until the client is able to accurately perform the procedure. Once this is achieved the client may extend the arm as fast as possible.

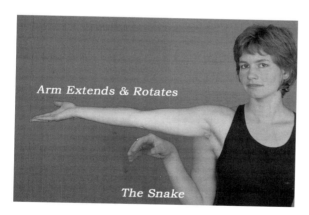

◀ *Figure 23*

NOTE: This extension must NOT be performed unsupervised. It is not an exercise to be continued after treatment.

CARPAL TUNNEL SYNDROME

The test for carpal tunnel syndrome is for the client to form a ring with the thumb and little finger. The therapist then attempts to pull the ring apart whilst the client resists. Any weakness or pain indicates that this procedure might be appropriate.

Carpal Tunnel Procedure Moves

The thumbs of both hands are positioned on the underside of the forearm. The thumbs then tease down the middle of the forearm firmly. This can be done more than once, leaving at least five minutes between each set of moves. When the procedure is completed, the arm can be 'closed up' by applying gentle inward pressure to the forearm, then the arm is gently stroked down from the elbow to the wrist.

Repetitive Strain Injury (RSI)

The so-called RSI can have extensor Moves 8 and 9 added for effect. As it stands, the reliance on habitual movement or work being blamed for RSI is something of a misnomer. The use of a keyboard by itself cannot and does not cause repetitive strain injury. There have to be other factors involved, including the angle and position of working, the height of the chair and more importantly the previous history of the client. Many clients who have a history of neck, shoulder or lower back problems can be predisposed to pains in the arms if a certain movement is applied.

In one case of a young tennis player diagnosed as having tenosynovitis pains in the forearm, her treatment consisted entirely of the upper back, shoulder and neck work. Her problem was resolved completely by this, as it transpired that she had been injured at an early age in the upper back area and this in turn had affected her arm.

HAMSTRING PROCEDURE

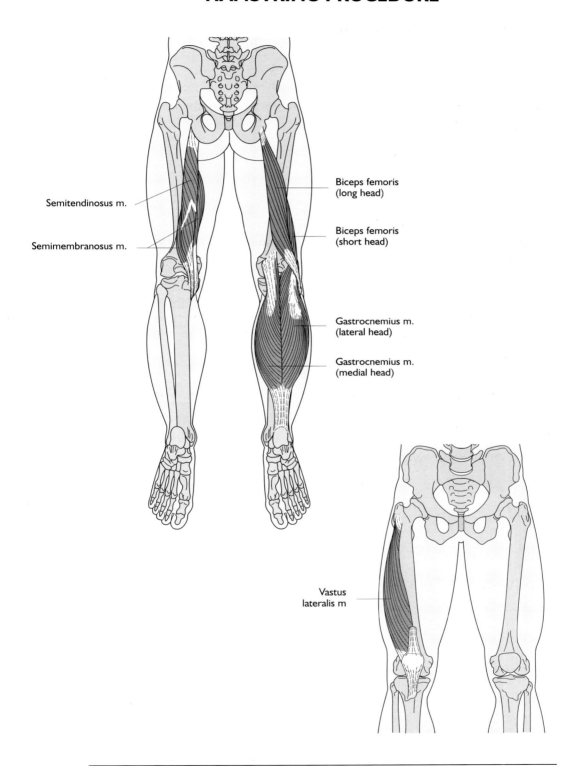

Semitendinosus m.

Semimembranosus m.

Biceps femoris
(long head)

Biceps femoris
(short head)

Gastrocnemius m.
(lateral head)

Gastrocnemius m.
(medial head)

Vastus
lateralis m

Muscles Worked Biceps femoris, semitendinosus, semimembranosus, gastrocnemius, vastus lateralis.	**Possible Indications for Use** Tightness or pain in the hamstring, knee problems, sciatic type pain, pelvic relaxer, to prevent sports injury and enhance performance.
In Conjunction with Other Procedures Page 1, pelvic, knees, ankles, TMJ.	**Cautions or Special Notes** Care should be taken with painful areas of the hamstring.

The hamstrings consist of four muscles, all of which attach to the lower edge of the pelvic frame at the ischial tuberosity, the sitting bones. Hamstrings are tough to get at because they tend to be covered by a good layer of tissue and they are also often tight and developed. The muscles that we are mainly concerned with are: biceps femoris, semitendinosus, semimembranosus, and gastrocnemius.

The hamstring procedure is an extremely useful one for people involved in sports injury. This area has always intrigued me, as I can't help but wonder why top athletes get injured so easily, when in theory they should be at the peak of their physical perfection. It seems that in a lot of cases there is little time to spend on prevention treatment and the focus is on 'repair and keep competing'.

The Bowen Technique has a powerful ability to prevent injury and due to its simplicity, even complete teams of athletes can be treated regularly and thereby avoid injuries that would otherwise occur frequently.

In addition to prevention, the hamstring procedure – along with certain other procedures – acts as a performance enhancer enabling all kinds of sports people to report that they perform to a consistently better standard. Perhaps this is due to a reduction in fear of injury or perhaps the fact that a hamstring will respond with a greater degree of flexibility after this work.

Observation and Assessment

Before beginning the hamstring procedure, it is important to assess if there is any major tenderness in the hamstring area. This can be done by applying increasing pressure with the thumbs, onto the long head of the biceps femoris, asking the client to indicate at which point any tenderness occurs.

Prerequisite Moves

Moves 1–8 Page One lower back are generally given before the hamstring is performed.

Hamstring Procedure Moves

Having done the assessment, the better side is treated first. In this example, better can mean less painful, or more flexible. The treatment for the left leg is as follows, with the patient prone.

With the right hand, the therapist picks up the left ankle and bends the knee to 90 degrees. This allows the biceps femoris muscle to be isolated and prevents the muscle from being contracted during the move. It is important that this angle is maintained to prevent tightening of the hamstrings during the procedure, as firm pressure will be applied. If the client is able to contract the biceps femoris even slightly, then this could be quite painful.

Moves 1–3. The therapists elbow is positioned onto the head of the biceps femoris with the arm at an angle of 45 degrees. After the skin slack is drawn

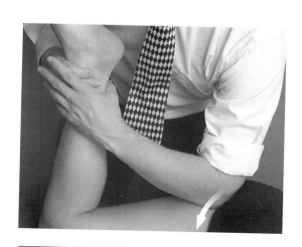

◄ Figure 24. Hamstring procedure Move 1.

laterally the move is made medially across the head of the biceps femoris, applying firm pressure with the elbow. Maintaining the angle at the knee, the left thumb makes a very gentle medial move across the popliteal fossa at the back of the knee. This is done in between the tendons at the back of the knee and not over them. Using the left hand to support the ankle, the ankle is rotated erratically with the right hand, after which a sharp downward blow is applied to the metatarsal ball of the foot with the little finger side of the therapist's fist.

These moves are repeated on the right side before allowing the hamstrings to rest for five minutes. This rest can be with the client prone or supine. During this break, if the client has been turned, other moves such as Page 3 neck can be performed. If not already turned over, turn the client after the rest and the lateral inferior border of the vastus lateralis is then moved medially.

The therapist stands with the back to the client, the client's leg is drawn up to a gentle angle, until the sole of his foot rests on the bed.

With the tips of the fingers midway down the inside of the leg, the two aspects of the hamstrings (biceps femoris and semitendinosus) are located. Keeping these two aspects clearly identified, the fingers walk down the middle of the leg towards the head of the hamstring group at the ischial tuberosity.

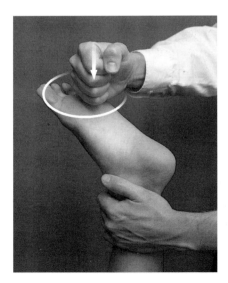

◄ *Figure 25*

CAUTION: It is important not to be invasive of the genital area. This can be prevented by bringing the forearm across to rest on the client's opposite thigh.

Moves 4–9. When the head of the hamstring group adjacent to the ischial tuberosity has been located, fairly firm pressure is applied and a move made medially over the head of the hamstring. Maintaining this firm pressure, a lateral move follows.

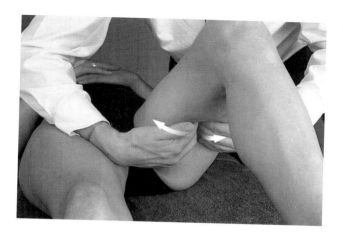

◄ *Figure 26. Hamstring Moves 4.*

Moving both hands to the middle of the leg and relocating the midpoint of the hamstrings again, the moves are the same as for Move 4, but with less pressure.

Using the middle fingers of each hand and starting in the middle of the popliteal fossa, just behind the knee, with very gentle pressure, the skin is moved medially and laterally. This move is a skin move, not going over the tendons either side of the popliteal fossa, but working in the small hollow at the back of the knee.

The therapist then moves to the foot of the client, sitting on the table with the client's toes wedged to prevent sliding. The tips of the fingers sit in between the medial and lateral heads of the gastrocnemius, approximately four centimetres down from the knee. A rolling move is then made around the medial and lateral heads of the gastrocnemius as for Moves 5 and 6 of the knee procedure. Moving down to the mid-calf, the separation of the gastrocnemius is repeated as for Move 7.

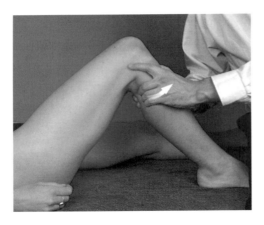

◄ *Figure 27. A rolling Move around the heads of the gastrocnemius.*

The Achilles is relaxed by gently moving across the tendon medially and laterally.

NOTE: To ensure that the hamstrings remain relaxed, gentle hamstrings stretches on a daily basis are recommended. Referral to a qualified teacher is advised.

THE KIDNEY PROCEDURE

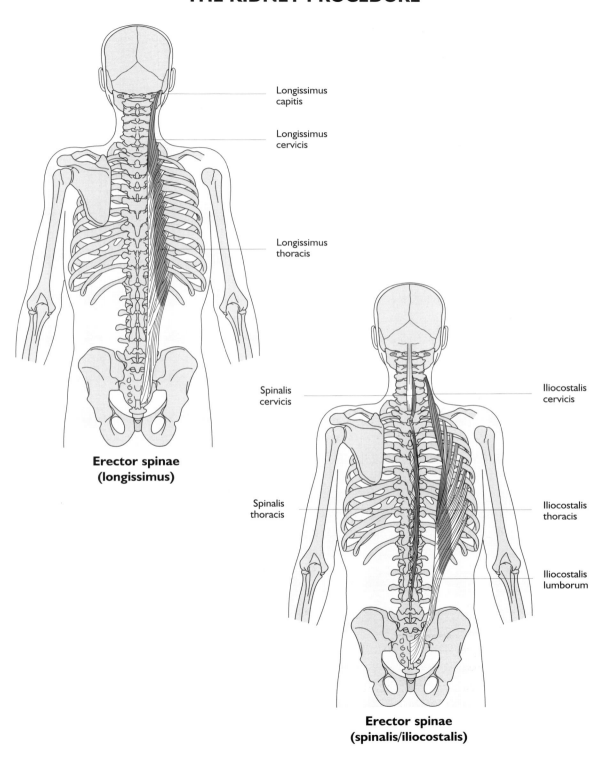

Longissimus capitis

Longissimus cervicis

Longissimus thoracis

Erector spinae (longissimus)

Spinalis cervicis

Spinalis thoracis

Iliocostalis cervicis

Iliocostalis thoracis

Iliocostalis lumborum

Erector spinae (spinalis/iliocostalis)

Muscles Worked Erector spinae.	**Possible Indications for Use** Nephritis, kidney stones, urinary tract infections, dialysis, low energy, ME.
In Conjunction with Other Procedures Stoppers, Pages 1 and 2, other lymphatic drainage procedures, pelvic, TMJ, breast.	**Cautions or Special Notes** Water intake must be good, especially following this procedure. Worse side treated first.

The kidney represents one of the more important areas of the adrenal system and one which takes a bit of a beating in the daily run of things. The glomeruli in the kidneys deal with something like 200ls of fluid a day that is filtered through. Fortunately most of this ends up seeping back into the system, but we can see from this the importance of a good water intake. Tea, coffee, alcohol are all diuretics, which irritate the kidneys and impair normal function if taken in excess and without adequate water.

For the purposes of The Bowen Technique, the kidney is one of the lymphatic drainage moves, of which there are four. Although not directly part of the lymphatic system, it is responsible for the effective removal of debris from the body. I always think of the lymphatic system as a sort of messenger boy cum sewage system, picking up accumulated tissue fluid and returning it to the blood circulation, whilst at the same time washing away dead blood cells, foreign substances and other unwanted bits and pieces. It also has an active part to play in absorbing fats from the small intestine, and for this relies on the right sort of fat in the diet. Another subject.

As you will expect, the move itself is a relatively simple one, in spite of the fact that it is working an area that can have a powerful effect on the system. The therapist should identify which kidney is the worst one and this can be done by assessing the temperature in the kidney region. A warmer side will generally indicate that this is the side that should be addressed first, the only exception to this being where one side is hot and the other cold. In this instance the colder side would be treated first.

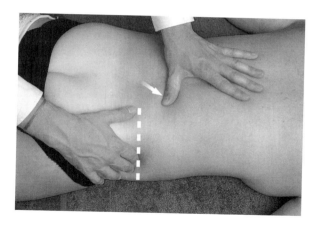

◄ *Figure 28. Position of the kidney Move.*

The Moves

The initial moves that will be performed before working the kidney area, are the lower stoppers, which are Page 1, Moves 1 and 2 and the upper stoppers, Page 2, Moves 1–4. These are followed by the middle section, Moves 9–12 which are pairs of moves performed either side of the spine. The amount of moves done here can be varied and in the case of a serious illness then it might be advisable to do none of the mid-section moves, but go straight into doing the kidney.

Having done these initial moves, the therapist decides which kidney is the worst one and stands on the opposite side. For example if the right kidney is the more affected side then the therapist will stand on the left. We will use this as our example.

With the right hand, the therapist reaches down and lifts up the leg by the medial side of the ankle and bends it to 90 degrees from the table. The leg is then allowed to drop out to the side of the client. This will generally be around 45 degrees but can be more or less. When the leg has dropped out to its own comfortable level, the therapist applies gentle pressure to the medial side of the ankle. This raises the opposite side of the body and presents the lower trunk to be treated.

With the left hand, the therapist locates the lower floating rib on the right side. Level with this on the erector spinae, the therapist makes an oblique and lateral move over the erector spinae, over the kidney. The move is made with the left thumb and directs the energetic effects of the previous moves towards the kidney. The left side is then treated. Although the left kidney is slightly higher than the right, the locating of the lower floating rib will still bring the move into range.

For aftercare, clients with weak or damaged kidneys or where there are kidney stones are advised in addition to water, to drink beetroot juice. This is from raw beetroot not cooked and no more than 25mls should be taken at one time. It should also be noted that this will show in the urine and the stools and appear bright red. Although not blood red, it can be quite a shock for someone to look into the toilet and see a brilliant colour looking back!

KNEE PROCEDURE

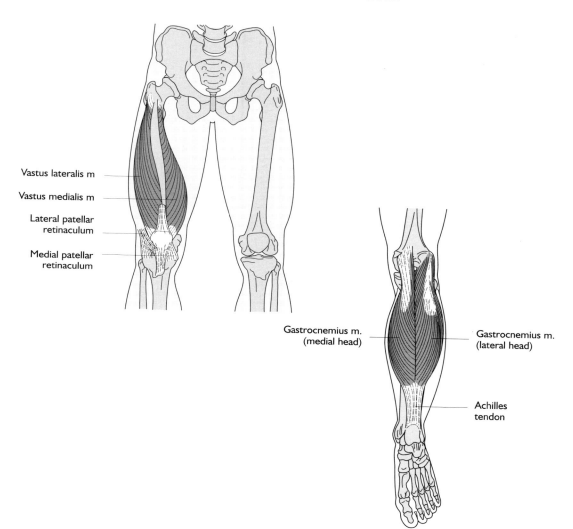

Vastus lateralis m
Vastus medialis m
Lateral patellar retinaculum
Medial patellar retinaculum

Gastrocnemius m. (medial head)
Gastrocnemius m. (lateral head)
Achilles tendon

Muscles Worked
Vastus lateralis and medialis, patellar retinaculum, gastrocnemius, Achilles tendon.

Possible Indications for Use
Ligament or tendon pain or damage, swollen knees, calf cramps or spasm.

In Conjunction with Other Procedures
Lower back (Page 1) pelvic, sacrum, hamstrings, ankle.

Cautions or Special Notes
The moves can be alternated from one knee to the other, i.e. left 1 – 3, right 1 – 3 and so on.

The knee is a complex structure with a myriad of jobs to do. As well as provide support for the body, it is required to make thousands of individual movements a day and take an incredible load. On top of this, the knee has only one source of lubrication, synovial fluid with which to make it all go smoothly. In terms of engineering it would be an impossible joint to reproduce.

A lot of things can go wrong with knees, and although the knee procedure is very useful it is definitely one that will be benefited by other procedures.

The knees will often be affected by other areas of the body particularly the lower back, but stomach, spleen and gall bladder are also areas which can affect the knee. Shoulders, which can often involve a knee problem, should also be considered in an overall assessment.

Prerequisite Moves

If unsure of a lumbar-related problem, the lumbar area should be addressed, using Page 1, Moves 1–8. As it will be generally impossible to be sure as to whether the lumbar area is affecting the knees, using the lower back work as a prerequisite to the knee procedure is advisable.

Knee Procedure Moves

Having completed the lower back moves, Page 1, the client should be turned to a supine position and the knee supported with a pillow if required for comfort.

Moves 1–3. The therapist moves the lateral inferior border of the vastus lateralis tendon medially next to the patella with the thumbs. This is the same move that is performed to complete the work done on Page 1, but in this instance also forms the first part of the knee procedure. The therapist then forms a grip with the fingers and thumbs on the fatty pad of tissue just beneath the knee cap, drawing skin slack and positioning the fingers and thumbs just underneath the patella. The therapist then moves the medial patellar retinacular fibres in an oblique medial direction with the index finger, rolling around the shape of the knee cap for Move 2 and immediately makes a similar move around the lateral knee cap in an oblique direction with the thumb for Move 3.

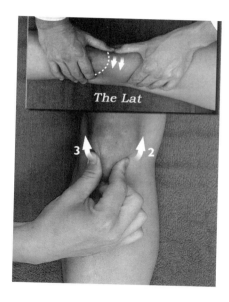

The Lat

3   2

◄ *Figure 29. Knee procedure Moves 1 – 3.*

Wait Two Minutes

Moves 4–6. The therapist finds the widest point of the vastus medialis approximately three fingers from the top of the patella and three fingers posteriorly. The skin slack is moved posteriorly and the move is anterior, made with both index fingers. This is a sensitive area and care should be taken not to apply too much pressure.

With the leg bent the therapist prevents any sliding of the foot on the bed, by sitting gently on the client's toes. The middle and ring fingers of each hand are positioned in between the medial and lateral heads of the gastrocnemius ensuring that the index finger of each hand does not touch the hamstring tendons or the popliteal fossa. After taking the skin slack medially the therapist makes a roll laterally over the lateral head of the gastrocnemius (see figure 27). This is repeated for the medial head. The medial head of the gastrocnemius is a different shape to the lateral head, resulting in a slightly different and less rolling feel to the move.

Wait Two Minutes

Moves 7–17. The medial and lateral aspects of the gastrocnemius muscle are then gently separated by moving down the calf with alternating medial and lateral 'teasing' moves. This is a very subtle set of moves and should feel pleasant and relaxing to the client.

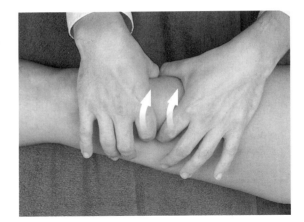

▶ *Figure 30. Knee procedure Move 4.*

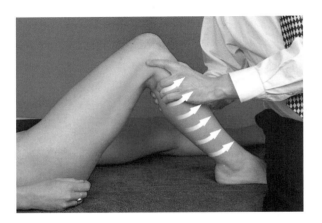

◀ *Figure 31. Knee procedure Moves 7 – 17.*

Three medial moves, 2.5 centimetres apart over the Achilles tendon finish the moves down the leg and create a drainage and opening. These teasing and Achilles moves, create an excellent opportunity for excess fluid to be drained from the knee and calf. Excess swelling in the knee will generally respond very well to the application of a washing soda pack, which can be applied two or three times per week on alternate days (see page 142).

Wait Two Minutes

Moves 18–22. Close the gastrocnemius by applying gentle pressure towards the midline of the gastrocnemius with either the tips of the fingers or by gently squeezing with one hand.

Move 22 is optional, which works at the base of the tibial bundle and affects the sciatic nerve. Useful for knee problems but also indicated in acute sciatic type pain. At a midway point between the peak of the medial malleolus and the Achilles tendon, move the tibial nerve and neurovascular bundle anteriorly.

No heat or ice should be applied to the affected area but apple cider vinegar (see page 141) can be used for inflamed or bruised knees, or where swelling and inflammation together are present.

Depending on the history of the condition, no exercise should be undertaken during the following week. This is an important element when treating knee problems. As with any injury, time will be needed but with knees there is an additional element of rest required, due to the load-bearing task of the joint. Running in particular is an activity that should be avoided after knee treatment, until any pain has eased.

PELVIC PROCEDURE

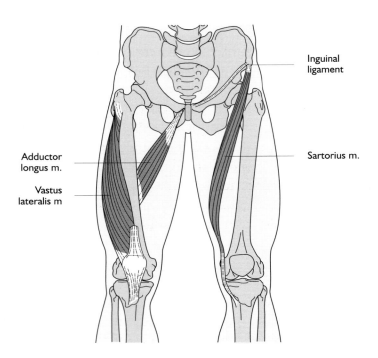

Inguinal ligament

Sartorius m.

Adductor longus m.

Vastus lateralis m

Muscles Worked
Vastus lateralis, adductor longus, sartorius, inguinal ligament.

Possible Indications for Use
Groin strain, hip problems, incontinence, leg length difference, general balance through the body. As a preventative for injury, especially sports.

In Conjunction with Other Procedures
Coccyx, hamstrings, knees, ankles, as part of a complete body balance.

Cautions or Special Notes
Works a possibly invasive area and should be done with thorough consultation with the client.

I am often laughed at by my students for regularly saying that every move would be the one that I would take with me to my desert island. If pushed I would have to say that the pelvic procedure would really be the one. Alongside the initial Pages of 1, 2 and 3 the pelvis would be the one procedure that I would most refer to in a clinical situation.

In many ways the theory of the pelvic is very similar to that of the coccyx. The three areas in the pie chart (see page 96) that we discussed with the coccyx are also very relevant to the pelvic. The main difference is that the coccyx tends to act as a powerful energiser whilst the pelvic acts as the physical balancer. So in the case of infertility for example, it is fine to energise the reproductive area, but if there is a physical imbalance which is tilting the pelvis, then it will be unlikely that a woman will be able to conceive, much less carry to term. This also applies to bladder problems. The coccyx will act as a terrific energiser to the bladder area, but if there is pressure on the bladder then this will affect the ability for it to function normally.

There is often talk of people having one leg longer than the other one and in my experience this is much rarer than a chiropractor will have you believe. Indeed there is a condition whereby the limbs grow at different rates, but this is extremely rare and for most people the cause of an apparent difference in leg length is a tilted or twisted pelvis. The exceptions to this are where there has been surgery such as a hip or a knee replacement, or perhaps where there is wear on a joint. Most of us however do have a tiny difference of as little as one or two millimetres and this is unlikely to cause much concern. The pelvic is another in the series of four lymphatic drainage procedures, due to the concentration of lymph nodes in the inguinal area.

The causes of a tilted or twisted pelvis are multiple and can be as simple as spraining the opposite ankle. Limping around for a couple of weeks will quite easily set up an imbalance which could in turn be present for years, causing all kinds of problems. Shoulder pain, RSI, irritable bowel syndrome and groin strain, are all conditions which can be caused or at least exacerbated by a moderately twisted or rotated pelvis.

The pelvic procedure has over the years amazed many manipulative therapists, who having assessed clients and re-assessed them after the procedure, have been stunned by how quickly the area has been affected.

Even more surprising however is that the work, once done, holds and does not need to be repeated, except in the case of re-injury.

The moves themselves are performed fairly high in the groin area and this procedure should be discussed carefully with the client before being performed. If the therapist has any concerns, then a third party should be present in the room.

Page 1, Moves 1–4 are the minimum moves that will be given as a prerequisite to the pelvic procedure.

Pelvic Procedure Moves

Turn client, having completed the prerequisite moves on the back.

The better side of the pelvis should be treated first or left side if unsure. To decide which is the better side, the therapist will initially ascertain from the client whether they have any pain on one side or the other. Treatment for right side: stand on the right hand side of the client.

Moves 1–4. 'Hit the lat'. With the thumbs, the therapist moves the lateral inferior border of the vastus lateralis tendon, medially next to the patella (see figure 29).

CAUTION: The client is asked to place his/her hand over the genital area and the therapist then covers the hand with a towel. The client must understand what is involved with the pelvic procedure.

Locate the anterior aspect of the adductor longus. With the index fingers crossed, the rest of the fingers of both hands are extended and the skin slack moved posteriorly following the shape of the muscle.

If the leg is bent to find the adductor then the right hand must lower the leg before proceeding with the second move. The adductor belly is gripped firmly for twenty seconds as close to the origin as possible (see figure 32), (the hand resting against the back of the client's hand) while the client takes two deep breaths. On the second complete exhalation, the therapist rolls anteriorly and firmly over the muscle belly. The client may now remove their hand.
A medial move over the sartorius is now made with both thumbs. The

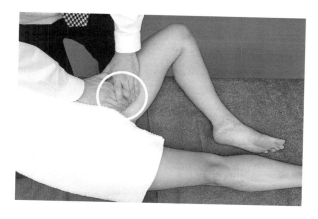

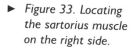

◄ *Figure 32. Move 2, pelvic procedure on the left side.*

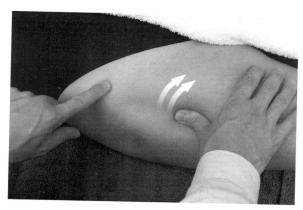

► *Figure 33. Locating the sartorius muscle on the right side.*

sartorius is located approximately 7–8cms inferior of the ASIS (anterior superior iliac spine) (see figure 33) and is the longest muscle in the body. Once again the position of the hands should be noted, ensuring that the therapist is not being invasive of the genital area.

With the index and middle fingers of the left hand apart and the rest of the fingers tucked into the palm of the hand, the therapist locates the inguinal ligament that runs from the ilium to the pubic bone. The two fingers then rest on the lower aspect (see figure 34).

The right leg is carried out 10–15cms and the knee brought to a slight bend with the sole of the foot on the bed. The therapist's right hand on the front of the knee pushes the knee across the body towards the opposite shoulder. At the same time a move over the now tightened inguinal ligament is made very gently, with the index and middle fingers of the therapist's left hand (see figure 35). As soon as the left hand has completed the move, the fingers are removed from this area and the knee continues to be pushed

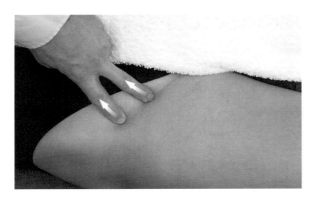

◄ *Figure 34. Locating
the inguinal ligament.*

towards the opposite shoulder, staying within the comfort zone of the client.

As soon as the knee has gone as far as possible, the leg is straightened and lowered to the table, being supported all the time. The opposite side is treated to complete the procedure.

CAUTION: Clients with hip replacements must NOT have their hip pushed through 90° at any time.

The client covering the genital area with his/her hand is a condition of performing this procedure, but must be preceded by an explanation.
Quite simply a miracle. Not just my words, but those of thousands of

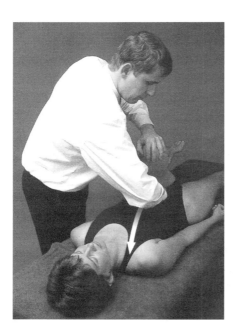

◄ *Figure 35. The therapist
completes the final part
of the pelvic procedure.*

SACRUM PROCEDURE

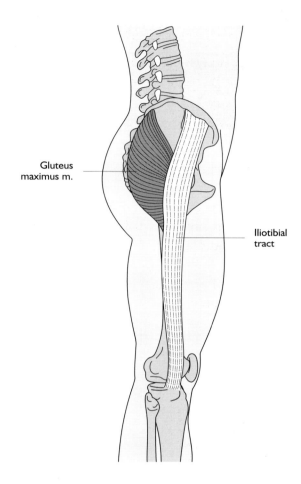

Gluteus maximus m.

Iliotibial tract

Muscles Worked Gluteus maximus.	**Possible Indications for Use** Acute lower back pain/spasm, back ache, period pains, back discomfort in pregnancy.
In Conjunction with Other Procedures Page 1, hamstring, pelvic.	**Cautions or Special Notes** The therapist should be aware of the hand positions, to avoid any invasiveness.

people who have experienced this procedure at first hand. I can't profess to be an expert on every other form of bodywork, but it would be difficult to imagine a procedure that is quicker than this and that has the effect that the sacrum procedure can have on a lower back.

The locked back is a common complaint and many of us at some stage will bend over to pick something up and experience that twinge which stops us in our tracks. For a lot of people however, it literally does stop them where they are, bent double and they will stay like that for some time unless they get some treatment.

Most acute back pain will go away eventually if left alone and given sufficient rest (as well as sufficient movement) but few people can be prepared to wait for this. The sacrum is the answer to this, and the number of people who have come in bent double with a solid back and who have walked out upright and pain free, will testify to the efficacy of this small couple of moves.

The moves are performed with the client standing and take a few seconds. This procedure is ideal for pregnant women and can be performed every day in pregnancy, to aid with back pain. Although the advice here is to give all the lower back moves before doing the sacrum, it is a move that can be done anywhere. Anyone with acute lower back pain can find that this procedure has the effect of a magic wand, in spite of the position appearing a little undignified!

Prerequisite Moves

Page 1, Moves 1–8 – observing the two-minute breaks as directed.

Observation and Assessment

Treat better side first or left if unsure.

Sacrum Procedure Moves

The client stands and leans on a table or the back of a chair.

The client should stand with their feet hip width apart and with their pelvis tilted forward. The lumbar region should be pushed out and the head lifted up. This exaggerates the presentation of the sacral region. The therapist stands on the same side being treated, ensuring that he can be seen by the client and is not standing directly behind the client. Treatment for right side as follows:

Moves 1 and 2. With the left thumb, the therapist locates the edge of the sacrum approximately two-finger widths lateral from the gluteal crease. The thumb should feel that it is resting on the margin of the sacrum, not on the actual bone itself. The skin slack is moved superiorly and then, applying firm pressure, the therapist moves inferiorly along the edge of the sacral bone with the thumb.

The hand is removed for a few seconds and then returned to its original location on the edge of the sacrum (see figure 36).
While the left thumb is holding on the edge of the sacrum as described

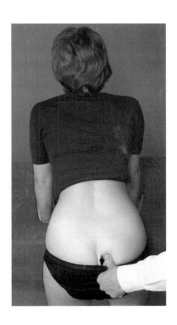

◄ *Figure 36. The thumb locates the sacral margin.*

above, the therapist's right thumb now locates the edge of the gluteus maximus and makes a posterior/medial move. This move is identical to Move 3 on Page 1, with the fingers resting on the upper part of the sacrum for stability and leverage. The left side would then be treated.

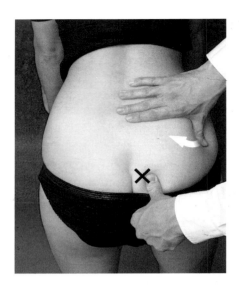

◄ *Figure 37. Move 2,
sacral procedure
slowly holding point.*

When the client stands, it is important to ensure that they stand evenly and don't tilt across onto one foot. The client has been leaning forward in order to take the weight off the sacrum and the sacroiliac joint. When they stand again, it is important that the weight is taken evenly so that the joint is effectively re-set.

NOTE: Whilst the sacrum and pelvic moves are complementary to each other, they may be performed separately.

The sacrum procedure can only be done with the client standing and is an ideal procedure for pregnant women that can be performed daily if necessary.

SHOULDER PROCEDURE

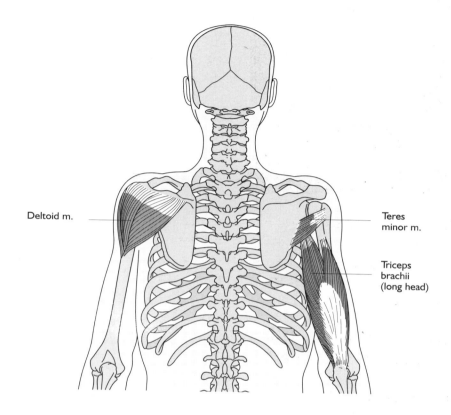

Deltoid m.

Teres minor m.

Triceps brachii (long head)

Muscles Worked Anterior and posterior deltoid, long head of triceps, teres minor.	**Possible Indications for Use** Any restriction or pain in the shoulder area, 'frozen shoulder', RSI, whiplash.
In Conjunction with Other Procedures Pages 2 and 3 upper back and neck as prerequisite moves, TMJ, elbow, pelvic.	**Cautions or Special Notes** Exercises are given with the shoulder. Any movement must be within comfort range of client.

The Bowen Technique boasts without doubt the simplest treatment for shoulders that can be found anywhere in the field of remedial therapy. Not only simple but highly effective, the shoulder procedure is rightly gaining a lot of attention, as a result of its ability to restore full range of motion and eliminate pain, in some cases instantly.

A research programme was commissioned by myself two years ago, which proved conclusively that not only was the shoulder treatment effective, but that the placebo element, often cited as a reason for complementary therapy being effective, has little part in outcomes.

Although the procedure itself consists of only two moves, there is the need when treating shoulder problems, to take a broad view of the client and look at other factors. There are of course the obvious elements such as neck problems and upper back symptoms, but then there is also a wide range of seemingly unrelated areas. Many clients that I see with shoulder problems also have: bowel complaints, knee pain, lower back pain or recent dental work, amongst others.

Moves 1–3

The shoulder moves are performed with the client upright, either standing or sitting. If the client is standing then it will be necessary to have an assistant who will carry the arm while the moves are being made. If working solo then the client will need to be seated. There have been suggestions that the work can be effectively performed with the client lying supine, but whilst this will give results in situations where only the deltoid is involved, it leaves a serious margin of error if there are other areas with problems. For this example we'll assume that we have an assistant.

Both shoulders must be treated in order to create a balance through the shoulders and upper back and the better or least painful shoulder should be treated first. After Pages 2 and 3 have been performed, the client is sat up and then asked to stand.

The assistant stands in front of the patient, holding the left elbow in the webbing of the right hand, just above the medial epicondyle. The patient's wrist rests across the assistant's left wrist. The assistant holds the arm at 35 degrees at chest height and ensures that the patient is relaxed and not tensing the arm.

The therapist positions his thumbs under the posterior border of the deltoid, on the axillary crease. The thumbs should be pointing to the ceiling with the skin slack drawn down (see figure 38).

On a signal from the therapist, the assistant starts to move the arm across the body. As soon as this starts to happen, the practitioner moves the posterior border of the deltoid quite sharply with a superior rolling Bowen move. The fingers at this time are resting on the top of the shoulder, acting as a lever for the action of the thumbs. The thumb move is made while the arm is in motion, being carried by the assistant.

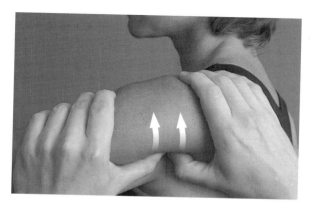

◄ *Figure 38. Preparing to do the 1st shoulder Move.*

The assistant should read this move on the triceps, in the webbing of the right hand. The reading of this move indicates that the deltoid and triceps have been moved and that the move (as opposed to the outcome) has been successful.

Once the reading has been registered, the assistant continues to carry the arm across the patient's body, continuing until the arm is locked over the

► *Figure 39. The assistant moves the client's arm across the body.*

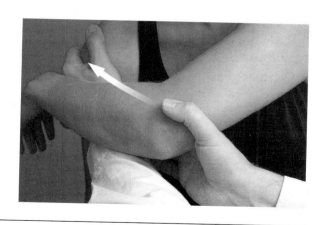

front of the patient. **THE ASSISTANT MUST NOT ALLOW THE ARM TO COME BACK EVEN SLIGHTLY**. The assistant will use their left hand on the patient's right shoulder to effect this close by squeezing the arm and shoulder together.

When the arm is completely across the body, the therapist jars the deltoid with the heel of her hand and only then can the assistant proceed to carry the arm back to the 35 degrees starting point.

With the arm in its original position, the therapist reaches over the shoulder with the tips of the index or middle fingers, rolls the anterior fibres of the deltoid superiorly and slightly laterally towards the coracoid process at the top of the shoulder.

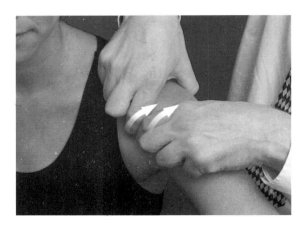

◄ *Figure 40. Second shoulder move.*

The shoulder may be treated again seven days later, but MUST THEN NOT BE TREATED FOR 28 DAYS. Other Bowen procedures may be executed during this time, but the 'no other therapy' rule remains in place. This is to allow the body to incorporate the changes that have been effected with the deltoid movement and is an important feature of the procedure.

TEMPOROMANDIBULAR JOINT (TMJ) PROCEDURE

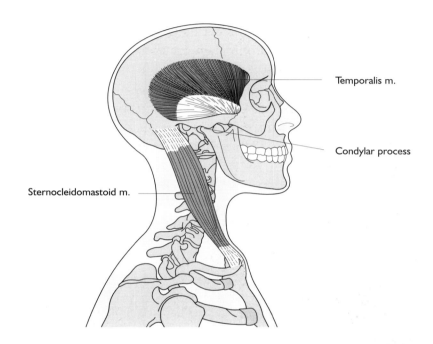

Temporalis m.

Condylar process

Sternocleidomastoid m.

Muscles Worked	Possible Indications for Use
Sternocleidomastoid, condylar heads of jaw, temporalis.	Extensive uses as a balancer and drainer for the face and head. As an adjunct to many Bowen procedures.
In Conjunction with Other Procedures Page 2 and 3 upper back and neck, asthma, shoulder, elbow. Other lymphatic drainage procedures.	**Cautions or Special Notes** A possibility of slight changes to the bite occurring and anyone with extensive dental restoration should be made aware of this. TMJ never performed with coccyx.

The TMJ procedure is, like the coccyx, a major balancing tool for the body. The areas that can be addressed by the TMJ is almost endless as it provides a structural reference point for the entire body. It is also one of the four lymphatic drainage procedures, providing an excellent form of drainage for the face and head, ideal for clients with sinus or hay fever problems.

Shoulders and RSI type problems respond very well to the TMJ, as it gives a balance to the upper back area and affects the nerves of the neck. All dental problems, including wisdom tooth compaction, bite differences, abscesses in gums, as well as many others can be addressed with TMJ work.

The lower back is one area that is often not considered when looking at TMJ but again the whole concept of structural balance relies on effective communication between lower back and the area around the inner ear. The stomach and colon are also assisted by the TMJ work due to the vagus nerve being located directly under one of the points in this procedure.

The caution with TMJ is that if a client has undergone extensive (and expensive) dental restoration, especially if this involves bridge work, then there is a possibility that small changes in the bite might occur, which may in turn affect the dental work. To this end, clients should be informed of this and given the choice as to whether to receive the work.

Prerequisite Moves

Page 2, Moves 1–8 upper back and shoulders, and Page 3, Moves 1–6 neck should ideally be performed before the TMJ.

Observation and Assessment

Drainage Moves 1–9. The therapist needs to locate the condylar fossae, slightly forward of the tragus, by asking the client to open and close the mouth. This is in order to feel the movement of the joint, and be able to visually assess the movement of the jaw and joint, observing any deviation or imbalance. This also 'sets up' the TMJ for later procedures.

On the midpoint of the mandible on its medial aspect, the skin slack is drawn posteriorly towards the angle of the mandible, gentle pressure applied with the middle finger and move made anteriorly along the line of the mandible towards the chin (*see* figure 41). A small lump or ridge can often be felt here, and this is the submandibular gland. Right side follows. At the level of the Adam's apple or thyroid notch, using the index finger,

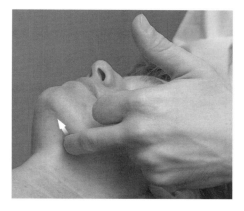

◄ *Figure 41*

the therapist draws the skin slack superiorly and moves inferiorly along the side of the larynx. Right side follows (*see* figure 42).

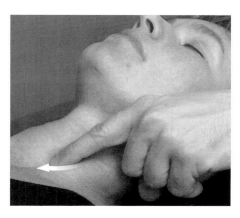

◄ *Figure 42*

At the left inferior sternocleidomastoid insertion, with the skin slack drawn laterally with the index finger, the therapist moves medially across the tendon. Right side follows (*see* figure 43).

By pushing on the lateral aspect of the trachea with the index and middle fingers from left to right, a slight click may be noticeable and this is the trachea moving across the hyoid bone. This action frees up the trachea and makes the subsequent drainage moves easier and more accessible.

The drainage of the lymph nodes behind the sternocleidomastoid (SCM) is

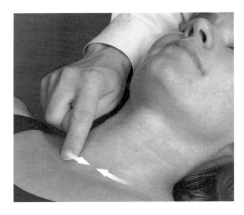

◄ *Figure 43*

now performed. Using the thumb and index fingers, the therapist creates a circle to pick up and enclose the SCM. The skin slack is drawn superiorly, gentle pressure applied between the thumb and index finger and a very careful move is made inferiorly. The drainage is started at the base of the throat and is carried on in small moves up to the mastoid behind the ear. The thumbs and fingers must not squeeze the muscle or allow it to slip from your grasp as this will be painful and potentially damaging for the client. Keeping the circle with the thumbs and fingers ensures that this is avoided (see figure 44).

When the therapist has reached the mastoid and can no longer grasp the

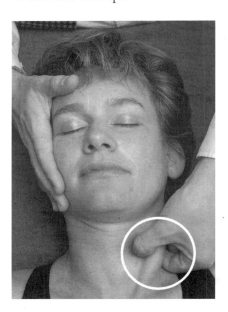

◄ *Figure 44. Drainage moves.*

SCM, the move is finished by pressing onto the belly of the SCM in a downward move.

With the middle fingers, the condylar heads anterior to the tragus of the ear are relocated on both sides. When satisfied that the correct position has been found, the client is asked to place the knuckle of one index finger in between the teeth and bite gently.

NOTE: Once the condylar heads have been located, the therapist must not remove the fingers or the heads will have to be relocated again.

TMJ Moves

1. Once the skin slack is moved anteriorly, gentle pressure is applied and a move made posteriorly over the head and joint.
2. Starting back on the condylar head again, the skin slack is this time taken superiorly, and a gentle inferior move is made over the head and joints. Moves 1 and 2 are performed on the left side before the right.
3. Locating the midpoint of the posterior border of the mandible, behind

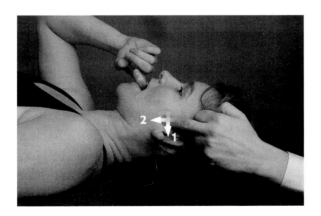

◄ *Figure 45. TMJ Moves 1 and 2.*

► *Figure 46. This move completes the TMJ procedure.*

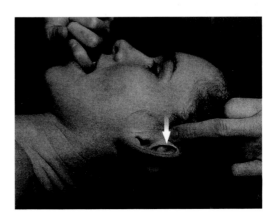

the ear lobe with the index finger, the therapist moves very gently inferiorly, along the posterior border of the mandible. A small lump can be felt here which is a point adjacent to the vagus nerve. Right side follows.

4. With the middle finger, a posterior move is made over the left temporalis muscle, located anterior to the edge of the ear and superior to the zygomatic process. Right side follows (see figure 46).

The therapist may then return and drain the SCM as before, noticing any changes that may have occurred. Drainage may be repeated at 5–10 minute intervals until the lymph nodes are no longer tender or restricted.

Chapter 5
Useful Remedies

Apple Cider Vinegar

Much has been written in the past regarding the use of cider vinegar as a medicinal tool. As well as outlining the use of it, I will also throw caution to the wind and say that as a remedial tool it outstrips the use of ice virtually completely.

Apple cider vinegar has been documented as being of use in a very famous nursery rhyme the origins of which are interesting and entertaining. Jack and Jill went up the hill to fetch a pail of water. Apparently Jack and Jill were doing more than fetching water and the village from whence they came was scandalized. When Jack fell down he actually broke his skull and the application of vinegar and brown paper was to no avail. Hardly surprising given the severity of the injury. And so the first documented failure of complementary medicine was seen. Although the story doesn't specify the type of vinegar used, the origins of it are from Somerset, where vinegar would be produced simply by allowing cider to 'go on'.

Cider vinegar is very different in its composition from that of malt or wine vinegars, in that it is alkaline-forming rather than acid. Its uses therefore are widespread but we are mainly concerned here with the treatment of soft tissue injuries. Cider vinegar acts as a negating agent for the acid environment of a sprain or muscle pull. Paula Esson, coach to the England women's basketball team, has been using cider vinegar extensively and has found it to be quite remarkable. She says:

"The use of apple cider vinegar in acute sports injuries to manage and reduce inflammation has been revolutionary on the court side. Marked reduction in pain and recovery time, has allowed players to return to the game fifty per cent faster than when traditional methods of heat and ice and have been applied."

Unlike ice, cider vinegar can be applied for long periods of time and has the effect of reducing pain and decreasing swelling rapidly. The application is very simple. A flannel or cloth is soaked in the vinegar and applied to the affected area. Some cling film or plastic can be wrapped around this in order to retain the moisture. In cases of sensitivity, skin can become red or even blistered. The vinegar pack can still be applied, but can be used diluted. Starting at 1:1 and going as far as three parts water to one part vinegar.

If there are any cuts or abrasions in the area then these should be covered with a smear of Vaseline in order to prevent the vinegar from penetrating and irritating the sore. Vinegar can be applied every day for one to two hours at a time and can also be taken internally for conditions such as arthritis, indigestion, tonsillitis, and as a prevention and cure for colds and flu.

Washing Soda

The humble washing soda crystal has all but had its day when it comes to washing clothes, with the advent of modern biological powders. For therapists however it still has several uses although it is becoming increasingly difficult to find in the shops. For our purposes we recommend its use for reducing swellings in joints, where no inflammation is present.

The action of the soda is that of drawing excess fluid from these areas, using osmosis as the principle for its effectiveness. Once again, it can be applied by the client at home as a pack which is attached to the affected area and left on overnight to work. As with the vinegar, any cuts or abrasions should be smeared with Vaseline, as even a small graze will itch terribly if the soda gets into it.

The soda crystals are crushed up to the consistency of coarse salt and placed in a handkerchief or similar piece of cloth, which is then folded up. The cloth must be cotton and the folded pack will measure approximately 10cms square. The folded pack is wrapped around the swollen area and secured with an elastic bandage. An old pair of tights will do just as well. The whole area must then be wrapped in a towel. It's not uncommon for anything up to one and a half cups of fluid to be drawn out of a swollen knee and this amount of fluid will make for a wet bed and an uncomfortable night.

In the morning the whole pack, soda and all, can be put in to the washing machine. If you are a massage therapist with oily towels, washing soda will break down the grease and restore your towels to their fluffy old self!

The pack can be applied every other night to a maximum of three per week. If the client does have sensitive skin, then they should try a patch test with one soda crystal under a plaster for twenty minutes to check for any reaction. One small note of clarification; the soda is washing soda not caustic soda!

Epsom Salts

Magnesium Sulphate or Epsom salts as they are better known, again battle with the acid that is responsible for the build-up of calcification in the joints. Anyone can use this method both as a treatment for painful, swollen or calcified joints, but also as a preventative measure for all of these. It's pretty good for bunions too.

Simply throw a mug full of Epsom salts into a bath whenever you have one. The softer your water the less you will need and you can still add oils or bath bubbles if you wish. Garden centres sell magnesium sulphate to put on hydrangeas, but this in my view is a waste of good Epsom salts. Most independent chemists will also be able to get it for you quite cheaply.

For smaller areas such as feet and hands, simply use a washing up bowl with about two tablespoons of salts per bowl. The water for this type of soaking should be warm and not hot and the soak should take around 15–20 minutes. If you are putting salts in the bath, be careful as it can make the surface very slippery.

Chapter 6
Research on The Bowen Technique

Researching the efficacy of Complementary and Alternative Medicine (CAM) has always been a somewhat difficult area, the result being that it is therefore comparatively rare. This is a stick used to beat CAM, which often cites the inability of CAM therapies to 'cure' disease and it is this cure which is the 'be all and end all' as far as many scientists and medical practitioners are concerned.

How often do we read: "There is no scientific evidence at all to suggest that whatever therapy works?" The very problem is one of the science itself being so narrow. A complementary therapist doesn't (or at least shouldn't in my opinion) treat specific disease, but should rather look at and treat the person afflicted. The result of treatment is that situations change and people's view of their own circumstances and illnesses change. The disease may or may not disappear, but that is not what we as CAM therapists set out to do.

Therefore to try and construct a protocol that examines a disease, a treatment and a group of people's specific reactions to that treatment, undermines the whole principle of what CAM is all about.

If someone walks into my clinic with a bad neck, I might look at his back, his knees or his jaw in order to help him. On the other hand, I might only look at his neck, but my view will be a broad one. To test this 'scientifically' is difficult. If I am to look at the efficacy of The Bowen Technique in the treatment of neck conditions, I must design a set of parameters that can be scrutinised. And yet the whole basis of the treatment is that we are not looking at one area or prescribing treatment for one particular problem.

To get around this I decided to set up a study programme, looking at the effects of The Bowen Technique on frozen shoulders. Since it is a relatively common complaint, I knew that it was one where even the basic moves had a good effect, even though the cause was often very multifactorial. In addition I wanted to challenge the widely held belief that any benefit derived from Bowen or other forms of therapy was purely placebo.

The Bowen Technique is such a light therapy, so what better way to test it out. In collaboration with Helen Kinnear, a sports scientist, we came up with a rigid protocol, together with a series of placebo moves and set about finding a group to practice on. After an article in the Sunday Times we were inundated with volunteers and eventually worked with a group of around one hundred, whittled down from literally thousands who contacted us wanting to take part.

The results were conclusive, with over **70%** of those treated showing an improvement, but at the same time there were some surprises. There was a benefit to those people who thought they were having Bowen but this benefit was not nearly as much as in those who were actually treated. The study was strict in its approach and insisted that the therapist could only perform prescribed moves, even if they saw that there was obviously another problem. In addition, advice to drink water and the exercises that we normally give, were omitted as it was too hard to monitor.

Further work with professional footballers is under way and a study is being conducted with other athletes examining the aspect of injury prevention using Bowen, compared with conventional treatment.

Research, as well as being time-consuming and expensive, can often be a diversion from what we need to be doing, but the absence of trials and studies can often be the stumbling block for many health professionals and state funded health centres.

The obsession with scientific outcomes is valid only if the science is broad enough to be inclusive, but currently is too rigid to be applicable to most CAM therapies. Evidence within CAM is the way forward and to this end I am currently devising a questionnaire which will seek to establish a percentile improvement ratio for all clients receiving a Bowen treatment. Over an extended period, I hope to show by sheer weight of numbers, that The Bowen Technique has a place in everyday treatment and is valid and financially preferable to many other conventional treatments.

Watch this space. In the meantime the summary of the frozen shoulder research programme is available on The Bowen Technique website: www.thebowentechnique.com.

In Conclusion

The future of soft tissue techniques such as The Bowen Technique has yet to be decided in terms of where they will fit into any modern health care set up. The system of administering drugs alone in order to treat disease simply isn't the answer, and as a result health systems all over the world are failing. They fail mainly because they view the patient as a disease, illness or injury to be treated, without looking at the welfare of the individual personality. It is an irony that in an age where cost is a key factor in determining availability of many drug treatments, the cost to society of overuse of drugs, in both financial and moral terms is incalculable.

Therapies such as Bowen offer an alternative, both in practice and approach. Instead of pursuing the goal of suppression and management it can surely be possible to explore the ability of the body to heal and repair itself. There is much that we do not know and possibly will never know about the workings of the human brain and therefore its dependent body and the need for everything to be scientifically proven is contradicted by how little we truly understand.

The Bowen Technique offers a bridge between the world of the medical doctor and that of the holistic approach. Certainly use drugs, painkillers, anti-inflammatories, surgery and other techniques, but first let us see whether the body has an answer for itself and whether from there, it is possible for us to promote health as an option.

In 2000 the health minister of the UK announced the good news that there would be more money spent on cancer – more surgeons, more hospitals, earlier detection. This we were assured would lead to a reduction in the number of deaths. It won't. The analogy is that of the Mayor of a town where the houses are all built of straw, and where the only source of lighting is candles, announcing that to deal with the continued house fires, he will be employing more firemen and building more fire stations. It's working at the wrong end and deals only with the problems rather than addressing the cause.

I would be the last person to suggest that The Bowen Technique is the answer to all our health problems, but what the approach represents could herald a major shift in the way that we view both disease and our attitude towards it. Surely it's worth finding out?

-The Bowen Technique
– Case Histories

The following case histories are included to demonstrate the power and effectiveness of Bowen. It's important to remember that although we are mentioning the resolutions to certain conditions, this doesn't create a blanket cure for all the named problems. Bowen treats the body as a whole, without referral to named disease, but naturally enough there are a lot of situations whereby presenting problems are resolved.

ANKYLOSING SPONDYLITIS OF THE LUMBAR SPINE

Man, aged 76   Ongoing treatments as needed

Diagnosis by GP: ankylosing spondylitis of the lumbar spine, confirmed by an MR scan. Mr G was in constant pain but refusing painkillers. He was unable to walk, without a walking stick, to his bank, which is only 5 minutes from his house. His GP said the only cure for the pain was an operation that could put him in a wheelchair. Mr G decided to try Bowen Technique. He had previously tried osteopathy, physiotherapy and acupuncture with little or no result.

He is a tall, slim man who was in obvious pain. There were no signs of muscle wastage. When he came for his second treatment, he was very much improved, walking without a stick. The pain was less, muscle tension almost normal, and range of movement improved. When he came for his third treatment, his movement was excellent, no pain, and very little pins and needles in feet. Since then, he has continued with a maintenance treatment once or twice monthly. He can walk around the town with no problems and no stick. He has remained pain-free for a year, apart from a slight hiccup when he walked his son's very boisterous dog, but this settled after treatment. He also had right knee problems 18 months after his first Bowen treatment but this settled after two treatments one week apart.

ANXIETY, NIGHTMARES, POOR CONCENTRATION, REPETITIVE MOVEMENTS

Girl, aged 9   5 treatments

A came with her mother, complaining of feeling anxious about school, having nightmares, difficulties with concentration, and making odd repetitive movements with her arms which other members of the family were finding irritating. Sessions one and two produced considerable improvement in general anxiety and behaviour. By the third session she looked much happier and more relaxed. School friends commented on how much better she was concentrating in class, and she found she was able to get on with schoolwork much faster. After five sessions, all odd arm movements had stopped; she was sleeping well, rarely having bad dreams.

ASTHMA ATTACK

Girl, aged 17   1 emergency treatment

England Junior Basketball Team Member, K, was involved with the multistage fitness test used to analyse an athlete's aerobic performance. A standard is expected at this level and the peer pressure to achieve the necessary grade is immense. K was struggling for breath soon into the test, causing some concern. Determination kept her going until she had to stop because she could not gain breath at all and had commenced a panic attack. K was removed from the concerned crowd and the Bowen emergency asthma move carried out. Immediately a normal breathing pattern resumed and after 30 minutes K carried on training with no further symptoms.

ASTHMA AND CHEST INFECTIONS

Girl, aged 8   3 treatments

F suffered with asthma and chest infections. She was small for her age and had a poor appetite. She had 3 inhalers: 5 puffs of one twice a day; 3 of another twice a day and the last one every 4 hours. Distressed with the amount of medication F was taking, her mother was looking for an alternative and discovered The Bowen Technique. After one treatment, F. became full of life, energetic, hungry and didn't need the 4-hourly inhaler. At the end of treatment 3, she was off all inhalers, had grown, was still full of life and hungry.

At a routine check up with the GP, just after Bowen treatment 3, he immediately picked up the difference. The bright, alert look in her eyes, weight and height gain, clear, good, strong breathing. He was so pleased he wanted Bowen information to give to other patients.

BACK: DEGENERATIVE DISC

Woman, 30s

B had pain in her lower and middle back with some spasm evident, plus stiffness around her shoulders. She had had a lower back injury as a child. She also suffered from stress. She had three children between 8 months and 4 years. She was moving house shortly after her second treatment. The pain in her back disappeared after the second treatment when the Bowen pelvic move was added and, despite carrying many heavy boxes during the move, she had no problems with her back. As the Bowen treatment is helping with her stress, this has continued.

In her own words:

"I have been diagnosed with degenerative disc disorder and have suffered for 12 years with lower back pain which has worsened since my children were born.

"All of summer 1999 the pain was severe and occurred frequently, often the pain going down into my legs and also up my neck and shoulder. After two sessions of Bowen it was almost completely better. Since then I had slight twinges, which have gone after a few days.

"In addition, the Bowen treatment seems to have had a marked effect on my general health, with practically no illness all winter, and also my mental/emotional health is much better. I don't have the down days and depression that I suffered for years."

BACK: CONSTANT LOWER BACKACHE

Woman, 40s   1 treatment

"I am a Consultant Paediatrician and, while my training has been in orthodox medicine, I have long been aware of the limitations of modern Western medicine in addressing basic issues relating to the promotion of health and well-being and prevention of disturbed function of the human organism. Over the last few years I have explored the preventive and therapeutic benefits of a number of practices complementary to medicine and have trained in several therapies. I was introduced to The Bowen Technique during a joint consultation with a kinesiologist who had trained in it. I had been experiencing a constant ache in my lower back for some time and therefore became the fortunate recipient of a Bowen treatment. To my amazement, I experienced immediate relief and this happy state held over time. I was so impressed that I enrolled in the training course and now also use The Bowen Technique on a number of conditions. If only The Bowen Technique could fit the criteria for acceptance in the current climate of Evidence Based Medicine, the benefits to individuals and the savings for the NHS would be enormous."

BACK: RIDING INJURY

Woman, 30s   several treatments

P had a bad fall from a horse 8 years previously and had been through back surgery in an attempt to correct the damage. This had not been successful, and after the surgery P received epidural injections for relief from the pain. At this point, she heard about The Bowen Technique and went to her local therapist. After just a few treatments, P was thrilled to be free of her back pain at last.

BACK PAIN & HIGH BLOOD PRESSURE

Woman, aged 54   3 treatments

Bowen Technique practitioner Annie Sewart, who is also a physiotherapist, treated Mrs C who came with a history of back pain, which included a particularly bad episode two years previously. Mrs C also looks after her disabled mother at home. Typically, her back pain would also travel down to her left knee. An x-ray revealed that 3 lumbar vertebra had reduced cartilage. Two weeks before she came for Bowen treatment, Mrs C's back "went" during a skiing holiday when she stood up from a sitting position. When she came for the first treatment, Annie noted that Mrs C also had high blood pressure. During the first treatment, Mrs C felt very woozy and was hot and flushed afterwards, so remained lying down for a while. She said that her back was then painful for two days following the treatment but that something "snapped" as she was walking and the pain was gone. At her third treatment, she reported feeling a bit stiff, but had been playing tennis. In addition, her blood pressure was normal for the first time in two years. One week later, she was feeling fine and has not needed further treatment.

BACK PAIN, RIGHT SIDE PAIN, & ASTHMA

Woman, aged 62   4 treatments

After her first treatment, M experienced a surge of energy lasting though the week and far less tension in her right calf, which had been virtually in spasm since an accident 9 years previously. She described her calf as 'melting'. After the second treatment she said, 'I cannot believe the difference in my back, almost 100% already'. Knee & hip pain were much lessened, and she was generally feeling much better in herself. She had cut back her asthma prevention medication. After the third treatment, she reported that the back pain she had had for 9 years (and had expected to always have) was now alleviated. She said she had no wheezing that week. After the fourth treatment she experienced one sore back day that cleared up by itself.

BELL'S PALSY

Woman, age 54   2 treatments

Mrs R writes: "On Friday, 1st September 2000, I was diagnosed with Bell's Palsy and was given a 5 day course of steroids and advised to see a neurologist. This would have probably taken several weeks with the NHS. I contacted Bowen practitioner Ron Simmonds on Monday 12th September.

"The symptoms of the Bell's Palsy were that my left eye had gone right up in the socket and the right side of my mouth had dropped so that I had great difficulty in drinking and eating.

"During the course of the first treatment, during one of the short breaks [that are a part of Bowen treatment], I could still feel movements around and under my left eye as though he were still working on it. When the treatment was finished, I looked in the mirror and was amazed to see that my eyes were symmetrical and back to normal. A week later I had a second treatment and my mouth showed a little improvement on that occasion. I had a third appointment provisionally booked for a week later but my face was so improved that I did not need it.

"I also had a private appointment with a neurologist on the 27th of September, by which time my face was completely recovered."

CERVICAL SPONDYLOSIS & ANXIETY

Woman, aged 68   3 treatments + monthly follow-ups

Mrs D has had cervical spondylosis for 5 years and suffers with tremors in her right hand. It also causes dizziness and pain in the back of her head. She was previously on anti-depressants for 3 years, prescribed after suffering with stress from work then a series of medical conditions including high blood pressure, a hysterectomy, pernicious anaemia and suspected cancer. She suffers with tension, anxiety, shaking and lip tremble and is very lacking in confidence, shy and retiring.

Mrs D felt wonderful after the first treatment and walked two and a half miles. After the second treatment, the pain had reduced and she felt 'good in spirits' and noticed an improvement in her piano playing. Her blood pressure was down and she managed to drink a cup of tea without shaking. After a third Bowen treatment she managed to drive a round trip of 400 miles and is gaining in confidence. She has continued to improve with monthly treatments.

FIBROMYALGIA

Woman, 30s   2 treatments

Following three years of fibromyalgia - worse in the past twelve months - G felt pain in her 'back, neck, limbs …all over'. After the first Bowen treatment she experienced extreme 'anaesthetic' tiredness for three days, then improved steadily: less pain, no falling down, almost no vertigo, and walking and sleeping better. After only two treatments other members of her support group also experienced real improvements.

GLUE EAR

Girl, aged 15   5 treatments

R came to see me recently with her mother. As an infant, from 1 year old, she had much trouble with glue ear, with resultant problems of hearing loss and weakness in speech development. At 4 years old she had grommets fitted, and the problem gradually resolved itself.

However, a bad head cold at 14 years started the problem again and her GP could only recommend specialist referral in 6 months time if there was no improvement. Mother and daughter were both very upset at the thought of having to go through "the whole grommets thing" again, and worried about the effects of a long-haul flight that R was soon going to have to cope with on the holiday of a lifetime to Barbados. R had 5 treatments with me before her holiday. She quickly started sleeping through the night for the first time in her life, and her mother reported that she had also started sleeping without making a lot of snorting and snuffling noises in her sleep, which she had done since a baby, and which they had both come to think of as normal. By the time of her flight she no longer had popping or discomfort in her ears, and her hearing was back to normal. I saw her after her holiday, and she had had no problems with the flight either way, and her hearing was still normal. I now see her every couple of months, to ensure she has no recurrence.

I.B.S.

Man aged 38   5 treatments

IBS had restricted P's lifestyle for over ten years. Not knowing when an attack might hit had left him almost house-bound. The first session with Bowen relieved the IBS but brought a lower back pain and a sore right knee to the surface. These were apparently old sports injuries from 15 years ago. The second Bowen exaggerated these pains further but the presenting IBS was not an issue. After five Bowen sessions all symptoms had been relieved and a full lifestyle maintained.

M.E.

Woman, 40s   regular treatments

"I have had ME for 15 years and like to think I know all its little tricks. I manage it reasonably well on a day-to-day basis as long as nothing too dramatic occurs in my life.

"1998 was to be the sort of year that would trouble most people. My father was terminally ill and I was flying to Bristol at least one a month, our house was up for sale and just ten days after his death, we moved. I think I worked through my grief by decorating the house from top to bottom over the ensuing 12 weeks. This would have been quite impossible under normal circumstances with ME but 1998 was not to be a normal year.

"In January I was introduced to a remarkable lady. Brenda Parker is a qualified Bowen Technique therapist. I cannot speak too highly of the treatment I am receiving from Brenda. I still have ME but it is easier to handle with the benefits my whole system has gained from this superb therapy."

MIGRAINES

Girl, aged 15   3 treatments

D is my own daughter. At fifteen years of age she was suffering from 3-4 migraines a week, usually waking in the morning feeling sick and unable to get out of bed until the attack had run its course. Life had become very difficult, and she was often off school till later in the day.

After only one treatment she had considerable improvement, and after three she had no more migraines. This improvement has held, and though she very occasionally has an "aura", she has not had another headache in the 18 months since treatment.

NECK: SEVERE RESTRICTION & LEG IMBALANCE

Man, 50s   2 treatments

Bowen practitioner Julian Wilson acquired one of his patients in an unusual way - while he was opening his business account at the bank and giving information about the nature of his business, the bank manager became so interested in the technique that he promptly booked in for a treatment. He was unable to move his neck, and one leg was 1.5 inches shorter than the other. He had been told that he would need a wedge under his left leg for the rest of his life. After only two Bowen treatments the bank manager had two even legs, a moveable neck and a lot of gratitude.

QUALITY OF LIFE - BLADDER CANCER

"Following a relapse into a second instance of bladder cancer, The Bowen Technique was recommended to me. Bowen practitioner Julian Baker agreed to treat me just as my chemotherapy course began and after only three sessions the effect was so noticeable that one of the chemotherapy nurses remarked that I was the most relaxed patient they had ever treated on that unit.

"The Bowen Technique therapy has dramatically reduced stress in both by body and in my mental attitude, removing old tensions and grievances to clear the way to a more balanced feeling now. The treatment has also considerably reduced the pain and physical problem of a frozen shoulder which had disturbed my sleep for months.

"In the space of eight weeks, Julian's application of the Bowen Technique to my body and problems has immeasurably increased the well-being I feel and, I am sure, has played a very important part in supplementing the conventional cancer treatment, to the extent that I now feel better than I have felt for over two years."

SPORTS: TRIATHLETE - SHINSPLINTS & PERFORMANCE ENHANCEMENT

Male, aged 26   2 treatments + 'top ups'

M was delighted with the results of the two Bowen treatments he received for his painful shinsplints. He decided to continue to have treatments on a regular basis because, he said: "I am now performing better than I have ever done before. In the past, I always managed to do very well in the training but on the big day I never seemed to be able to match my training performance. However, now, I am actually achieving far higher placings than I have ever done before."

He puts this sustained improvement down to The Bowen Technique and continues to come for regular treatments because he believes that not only is it a performance enhancer but that it is also a preventative to injury.

CEREBRAL PALSY, QUADRIPLEGIC

Bowen practitioner AC has used The Bowen Technique to good effect in the treatment of her son, C. She has produced this very informative, sensitive and thorough study of the effect Bowen has had on C. and we thank them both for allowing us to share it here.

Date of Birth - 8.10.88
Diagnosis: Quadriplegic cerebral palsy with athetoid features, markedly worse left side
Ataxia.
Deaf in left ear.
Visual problems.
Complex partial seizures.
Left leg one inch shorter than right.

How Does It Affect His Life?

Left side of body slow to respond, weak and poorly controlled.
Movements generally clumsy, balance poor.
Left leg splinted to prevent inversion of foot due to hypertonic tibialis posterior. 1 cm raise.
Left leg inwardly rotates from hip.
Poor motor control gross and fine.
Migraine headaches with vomiting on average twice monthly.

Emotionally C has mildly compulsive behaviour, high anxiety levels, is immature for his age and has poor social skills

C. is often confused, his thinking processes are slow, his concentration is patchy and he is highly distractible.

C. finds difficulty in instigating any action, or using his own initiative.

He worries a lot, has occasional 'turns' when he is 'absent' for a short time, and is frightened of being on his own.

He is frightened of going to sleep, cannot sleep on his own and often wakes at night.

He can't ride a bike except a specially adapted one, but would love to.

Treatment

I started very slowly with C. He has a lot of things to cope with and I felt he might turn against treatment if I did too much too soon. We started 2 - 3 weekly with P123. He enjoyed the treatment (he has not always enjoyed other therapies). Soon he was requesting treatment. "I think it helps me", though he was not able to say how. During treatment he would very quickly become quiet with a slow blink rate, often after only the first two moves were put in.

His whole system felt incredibly jumpy and irritable during treatment - some moves would make his whole body shake, or set off involuntary movements in limbs. Notably the left shoulder move and left vastus lateralis. This has become less marked as time has gone on. His whole system seems calmer now than when we started about 7 months ago.

At present, I treat whenever C. requests, usually about weekly, but I do the ankle procedure every day after exercises and before putting on his splint for the day. I may repeat it in the evening when I have taken his splint off. Often I will tuck a short treatment in when C. asks for it so we do not have to make too much of a performance, and sometimes I will pop in the usual first moves if he is lying on the floor watching TV, etc.

What Treatment?

Anything and everything! Often he will have some idea what he wants and will ask for a pelvic or a TMJ (temporo mandibular joint move) himself. Otherwise, I will rotate treatment, or choose according to where he seems to be having problems at that time. Hamstrings are a problem as he cannot stop giggling because it tickles but otherwise he enjoys all treatment.

Are There Any Changes?

Yes, without doubt. Almost immediately we noticed changes in C on an emotional level - he seemed brighter, more awake, more inclined to initiate actions, less troubled, dropped asleep more quickly and slept more soundly. Concentration at school improved, and some of his compulsive behaviours were less noticeable and less frequent. Visiting family members who had not seen him for a while commented on the change. Staff at school commented too, and they had not been told he was having any therapy. One family member described him as seeming more 'normal', and that just about says it all.

Gradually other changes are becoming apparent on a physical level. Since adding the pelvic procedure, C is walking better with less inward rotation from the hip. His ankle is making good progress and remaining loose enough to put plans for botulinum injections or surgery on hold. Orthopaed's comment - "Well, something must be working". He is using his left arm more and with improved control, his swimming style has improved and he can now manage 11 lengths in a session.

These are all small changes that together make a lot of difference to C's life - and ours. Very importantly, C enjoys treatment and feels it does him good. In this respect, I am sure he knows much more than we do and other changes may well become apparent. A journey of discovery and hope.

Useful Resources

ORGANISATIONS

ECBS
38 Portway, Frome,
BA11 1QU
Tel/Fax: 01373 461873
e-mail: info@thebowentechnique.com
www.thebowentechnique.com

Contact ECBS for more information
about The Bowen Technique and
training courses in the UK, Europe
and USA.

BTER
(Bowen Therapists' European
Register) PO Box 2920, Stratford
upon Avon, CV37 9ZL
Membership enquiries: 07986
008386, General enquiries: 07986
008384. e-mail: info@bter.org
web: www.bter.org

The Bowen Therapists Federation of Australia
www.bowen.asn.au/serv01.htm
Brian Smart Tel: 08 8584 5998;
Libby Gordon Tel: 03 9809 0688

For details of therapists and courses in
Australia and New Zealand.

The Nutrition Society 2001
10 Cambridge Court,
210 Shepherds Bush Road,
London, W6 7NJ

Tel: 020 7 602 0228
e-mail: office@nutsoc.org.uk

BOOKS

Atlas of Skeletal Muscles
Robert and Judith Stone
ISBN 0 07 116992 X,
McGraw-Hill Higher Education, New
York

Mosby's Basic Science for Soft Tissue and Movement Therapies
Sandy Fritz, Kathleen Maison
Paholsky, M. James Grosenbach
ISBN 0 323 00284 6, Mosby

BMA Guide to Drugs and Medicines – new edition each year
or more regularly.

Super Therapies
Jane Alexander – contains a very good
article on Bowen.
ISBN 0 55340 997 2, Bantam Books
£6.99 (NOW OUT OF PRINT –
possibly available from used book
search – see MC
Books, below)

Your Body's Many Cries for Water
F. Batmanghelidj, MD
ISBN 0 95309 216 X,
Tagman Press

Body Control the Pilates Way
Lyn Robinson
ISBN 0 33036 945 8, Pan

Gesundheit!
Patch Adams, Maureen Mylander
ISBN 0 89281781X,
Healing Art Press

BOOKSELLERS

W & G Foyle Limited
113–119 Charing Cross Road,
London, WC2H 0EB
Tel: 020 7 437 5660
Fax: 020 7 434 1580
General bookseller. Largest
independent stockist in the UK.

Houghton's Books
42 Victoria Avenue
Chard, TA20 1HE
Tel: 01460 67950
Specialist mail order bookseller
of medical books.

MC Books
21 Upper Bognor Road,
Bognor Regis, PO21 1JA
Tel: 01243 868614
Out of print book search.

Osteopathic Supplies Limited
70 Belmont Road,
Hereford, HR2 7JW
Tel: 01432 263939
Specialist mail order bookseller
of medical books.

Russell Medical
PO Box 3, Hanley Castle,
WR8 0DJ
Tel: 01684 311 444
Fax: 01684 311 555

e-mail:
thetallguy@russellmedical.co.uk
Specialist bookseller of
medical books.

NEWSLETTERS

**What Doctors Don't Tell You
(professional newsletter)**
Satellite House, 2 Salisbury Road,
London, SW19 4EZ
Tel: 020 8 944 9555
Fax: 020 8 944 9888
e-mail: wddty@zoo.co.uk

Informed Parent Network
For information on vaccination.
P.O. Box 870, Harrow, HA3 7UW
Tel/Fax: 020 8 861 1022

Soil Association
Organic information and
excellent newsletter
Bristol House, 40–56 Victoria Street,
Bristol, BS1 6BY
Tel: 0117 929 066
Fax: 0117 925 2504
e-mail: soilassociation@.org.uk

PRODUCTS AND SUPPLEMENTS

Biocare Nutritional Products
Technical support and free
seminars for practitioners.
180 Lifford Lane,
Kings Norton, Birmingham,
B30 3NU
Tel: 0121 433 3727
Fax: 0121 433 8705

**Colloidal Silver and Colloidal
Silver Machines**
Naturals at Earth Force,
1 Upper Belmont Road,

Bristol, BS7 9DG
Tel: 0117 904 9930
Fax: 0117 904 9931

Living Energy Systems
PO Box 37,
Totnes, TQ9 7YS
Tel/Fax: 01803 812332

Chlorella Products
Suppliers of chlorella,
anti-oxidant (AO3), wild yam
and colloidal minerals, etc.

The Barn, Sheppard's Farm, Draycot
Foliate, Swindon,
SN4 0HX
Tel: 01793 741122
Fax: 01793 741133
e-mail: sales@chlopro.demon.co.uk

Higher Nature
Suppliers of colloidal silver,
flax seed oil, lycine and
vitamin C.
For information and full products list
contact:

Burwash Common,
East Sussex, TN19 7LX
Tel: 01435 882880
Fax: 01435 883720

Savant Distribution
Suppliers of supplements,
FMD herbal products,
Udo's choice oil, etc.
Quarry House, Clayton Wood Close,
Leeds, LS16 6QE
Tel: 08450 606070
Fax: 0113 2745777
e-mail: info@savant-health.com
web: www.savant-health.com

HORSE BOWEN

Beth Darrall
9 Byron Road, Cheltenham, Glocs,
GL50 2PD
Tel: 01242 251465
Mob: 07759 439713
e-mail:
beth@equinebowentherapy.com
web: www.equinebowentherapy.com

Index

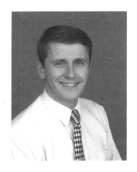

About the Author

Julian Baker is Europe's most experienced teacher and practitioner of The Bowen Technique, having brought the technique from Australia in 1992.

Julian Baker was born in London and after leaving school, had a successful career as a chef, training at Langan's Brasserie. In 1987, he and his wife embarked on what was to be a two-year trip around Asia and Australia. However, when they arrived in Queensland, they both quickly decided that they would apply for residency and subsequently citizenship.

Julian started to study reflexology whilst working as an executive chef at a large resort and was then introduced to The Bowen Technique in 1988 via a chronic neck problem. After moving to Brisbane, Julian started to practice Bowen and reflexology from his home, before returning to the UK in 1992 with the intention of introducing Bowen to the UK.

After two difficult years, a journalist for the Daily Mail wrote a large piece on the technique and the response was overwhelming, with over 5,000 letters arriving in two weeks. Julian and his wife Louise, subsequently continued in the promotion and education of Bowen, forming an independent therapists organisation in 1998, the Bowen Therapists European Register (BTER).

Julian lectures all over Europe and has recently set up an extensive teacher-training programme, the only one of its kind within the field of Bowen. A practicing Buddhist and keen golfer and squash player, Julian has two children and lives in North Somerset.